Closing the Circle

True Stories of
Navigating End-of-Life Care

Written for Healthcare Providers
by Healthcare Providers

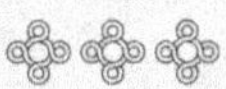

Inspired by the work and career of
Gail Daly, PhD, MSA, RN

Ann Caulfield-Cook, PhD, LMSW

Martha Hnatiuk, MA, RN

Chapbook Press

Schuler Books
2660 28th Street SE
Grand Rapids, MI 49512
(616) 942-7330
www.schulerbooks.com

Closing the Circle: True Stories of Navigating End-of-Life Care Written for Healthcare Providers by Healthcare Providers

ISBN 13: 9781966196532

eBook ISBN: 9781966196556

Library of Congress Control Number: 2026900733

Cover photograph (approaching sunset over Lake Michigan, Manistee, MI 2025) by Wendy Lineweaver

Editing by Dana Dunham

Printed in the United States by Chapbook Press.

This book is dedicated to

the patients who profoundly shaped my
perspective of end-of-life care

the families who loved them

and all the healthcare providers who understand
the significance of closing the circle.

Gail Daly

Note to Readers

Closing the Circle is an account of events that took place at Oakwood Hospital in Dearborn, Michigan, from 1989 until 2012. Oakwood Hospital merged with Beaumont Hospital in 2014. Beaumont has since merged with Spectrum Health and became Corewell Health in February of 2022.

The stories in this book are true, but the patients' names and identifiers have been changed.

Gail had many conversations and connections with healthcare providers throughout her career. They are not all included in this book, but each was instrumental in supporting end-of-life care and resolving ethical conflicts.

Closing the Circle is not a comprehensive study of end-of-life care or medical ethics and is not meant to capture the whole scope of these complex and nuanced fields. Instead, its purpose is to share lessons that will help inform healthcare providers about the challenges and rewards of end-of-life care, and to promote discussion and reflection about the role they play in assisting their patients in closing the circle.

Table of Contents

Preface

Gail Daly, PhD, MSA, RN, thrived in the fast-paced environment of the ER. She also flourished in critical care units on the medical floor, soaking up every new technical nursing development like a sponge.

But Gail really excelled at developing personal relationships with her patients, offering them warmth and compassion at difficult times in their lives. Like all medical professionals, Gail went into the field to save lives—but she found that it was helping patients at the end of their lives that held the most significance for her.

She often witnessed firsthand the turmoil that end-of-life events caused patients and families in the critical care unit of a hospital in the 1990s:

> At that time, visiting was very limited in critical care. To me, this was wrong. It was completely wrong, and I fought hard to allow visitors. The whole communication thing became very important to me. I could see the need for it in the family's faces when I would go out personally to update them in the waiting room.
>
> I remember we were doing CPR on a patient. His heart was failing. The resident would go out to the family and say, "Do you want us to keep going?" The family would say, "Of course we do." I followed the resident to the waiting room the second time, and he asked the same question: "Do you want us to keep going?" I said to myself, *Wait a minute. They need to hear what is going on and see what is going on.* I told them I would take them to the hall where they could see the room…They insisted on seeing the patient, and so I took them around the corner to bed 18. There was a lot of activity going on. It didn't take them two seconds before they said, "My god. Stop. That is enough."

Gail categorized the end-of-life cases she was involved in as "the good, the bad, or the ugly." What was the difference between them?

In most cases, the deaths that fall into Gail's category of a "good death" do not depend on the patient's disease or length of illness, but rather on whether the patient's integral beliefs and values have been identified and serve as guidelines for the decisions made in the patient's last days. These decisions may involve family communication, supportive interventions, ethical considerations, and sharing a true picture of the medical prognosis.

While end-of-life experiences may vary greatly among patients, a "good death" is one where the person who is dying has been heard and understood, and the choices that are made for his or her end-of-life care reflect this understanding.

Gail spent more than 40 years working in hospitals as a nurse and administrator. Through it all, she was guided by a mission to help patients, and their families, experience a good death.

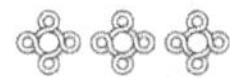

Closing the Circle offers the collective wisdom of Gail and her colleagues who committed themselves to helping patients experience good deaths. It is Gail's story, and also the stories of those who worked alongside her and supported her efforts. They include physicians, ethicists, chaplains, advance practice nurses, staff nurses, an attorney, a social worker, and a clinical diversity and language specialist. Despite their different backgrounds and specialties, they were all deeply affected by Gail and her dedication to improving end-of-life care.

Mohammad (Moe) Rustom, MSA, RN, FACHE, was an ER nurse who became part of Gail's crew in the early years:

One day Gail was walking around with her other nurse staff member, Chris Westphal. They were looking for a new staff member for Family Matters, and they stopped me and talked to me. They watched me and scrutinized me a little bit and later told me they thought…*this guy looks good*. The next day Gail came back, and she asked me, "Can you come up for an interview so we can sit down and talk?" She later told me the job was mine if I wanted it.

When Moe agreed to join Gail, he changed the trajectory of his career.

Ann Caulfield-Cook, PhD, the social work supervisor at Oakwood, was also recruited to the department after she was approached by Gail and clinical nurse staff member Martha Hnatiuk:

When Gail and Martha approached me to work in the ethics department with them, I knew I could not say no. I was shocked when they approached me and unaware they had their eye on me and my work. It was an exceptional compliment to be included in that sphere of people working in ethics and on the ethics committee.

Gail carefully selected these and others for her mission. She had a knack for recruiting the right people. It was something she had a gut feeling about, an instinct that picked up on a person's genuineness or sincerity. She wanted hard-working, dedicated people who recognized the importance of family. People who were tough enough to do the right thing for the patient. Those willing to stand up to any opposition they might encounter when honoring a patient's wishes and committed to following ethical principles no matter what resistance might arise.

With the team she assembled, Gail developed protocols that helped Oakwood navigate end-of-life case scenarios and established policies for withdrawing treatment, identifying non-beneficial treatments, and documenting end-of-life wishes, as well as guidelines for code status and accommodating patients' spiritual and cultural integrity. She even co-authored the hospital's award-winning advance medical directive document, *My Voice - My Choice.*

Closing the Circle is a tribute to Gail and the compassion and guidance she offered to her patients, their families, and the staff who cared for them. It is an exploration of her achievements in helping patients and their families find a wholeness at the end of life, despite their sadness and disbelief. It is an attempt to capture the wisdom Gail earned while she participated in countless end-of-life journeys—and to offer it to you.

As healthcare professionals, we play an important role in our patients' end-of-life experiences. While our training is in the sciences, our role in helping our patients close the circle of their lives is an art. It is not unlike a dance we join in together until the final notes make the song complete. It is a dance you and your own loved ones will one day participate in, a closing of your own circles, that may be better accomplished by what you will learn—by what we've all learned—from Gail.

Chapter 1

Gail's Journey

Do not go where the path may lead. Go instead where
there is no path and leave a trail.

—Ralph Waldo Emerson

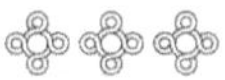

Gail Daly started her career in healthcare as a "candy striper" volunteer. In the years that followed, step by step, she became a champion for a patient's right to self-determination, and she developed a deep understanding of the end-of-life experience.

We have known Gail for many years, but as we interviewed her to collect the many lessons she learned over the course of her career, we were amazed by all that she had accomplished. She came up against many challenges, both personal and professional. But whenever Gail had a goal in mind, she approached it with determination and diplomacy and she always found a way to get it done. By sharing her story with you, we hope to show you how her work improved the lives and deaths of so many, and to invite you to think and talk about how Gail's experiences might help you assist patients in achieving a "good death."

Critical care nursing takes a certain type of person—one who can endure multitasking, adrenaline rushes, and crises. Gail Daly was born to be a critical care nurse. A diminutive woman at 5'3" and under 120 pounds, she was a ball of energy in the emergency room and on the critical care floors where she worked. In addition to taking on a high-stress nursing career, she was a single mother of two daughters who never shied away from a challenge. Whether it was skydiving, scuba diving, practicing and teaching martial arts, fostering three high school students, or completing her PhD while working full time, she took things in stride.

Gail's career path went from the Cardiac Care Unit (CCU) staff nurse to CCU head nurse. She eventually co-created the Family Matters Support Service (FMSS), which was dedicated to improving communication among patients, families, and healthcare providers. Gail then became a co-chair of the hospital's System Clinical Ethics Committee (SCEC) and Director of the Clinical Ethics Consultation Service (CECS).

Her decades of work with critically ill patients, their families, and her healthcare colleagues taught Gail many lessons about end-of-life experiences.

She learned what it was like to reach into an open chest, grasp a failing heart with her own hands, and pump blood through it until her arms grew weary.

She learned how to guide patients through the steps of completing an advance directive, saving them from treatments they never would have wanted by helping them find their voices to convey their wishes to loved ones—while they were still able to do so.

She learned from patients' family members who understood and accepted when heroic resuscitation efforts were not working, and from those who could never find the voice to say, "Stop. Enough."

But Gail's journey was not only professional.

She also learned from her own firsthand experiences with the death of her parents, one a peaceful death and the other a tormented one. Even after she retired, she continued to care for those who were closing the circle, nursing her partner of almost 40 years until his death in the home they shared.

Gail's lifelong journey taught her profound lessons about what it means to have a good death. Her journey began when she was saving lives in the emergency room.

Skill and speed in the emergency room

Gail's nursing career began in 1965 in an adolescent psychiatric intensive care ward in Michigan. But a divorce prompted her to change her life, and with her two young daughters in tow she moved to the busy city of Jacksonville, Florida, where she started working in an emergency department.

In Jacksonville's ER, Gail needed to move rapidly from one gurney to the next, wrestling drug addicts with stab wounds, or finding a crucial vein in an infant in distress. Most cases revolved around implementing lifesaving measures for major trauma, such as gunshot wounds and auto accidents. In these situations, all hands were needed on deck, and she was part of a team that had the specific goal of stabilizing those in a medical crisis.

The ER is about saving a life by any method available. But Gail was becoming attuned to a different sort of vital sign.

During her work in the ER, Gail always had a hemostat clamped to her uniform and ready for use:

> I have a pair of hemostats that I've owned for many, many years. I just saw them the other day in my drawer, and it reminded me of the story of an elderly gentleman I took care of when I was a trauma nurse. He was 95 years or older. He lived in a nursing home and had some dementia and was very, very agitated. I was changing his IV, and I always wore my hemostats clipped to my scrubs. As trauma nurses, we always kept them handy.
>
> While I was getting his blood pressure, I leaned over him, and he was kind of in and out of it, and he started

grabbing the hemostat. The nurse that was there said to me, "Stop him from doing that!" But I said, "No, he's fine." He kept grabbing, and I finally asked him: "Do you want to hold them?" I thought maybe he wanted to hold them. So, I put them in his hand, and he actually put his fingers in the little holes, and I heard it go click. He knew how to work them. I told him: "You can hold on to them for as long as you want."

The nurse was telling me, "He could poke you with that!" I said, "No, look at the smile on his face," as he was holding the hemostat. I looked at my stethoscope and said, "Do you want my stethoscope too?" Then he grabbed the stethoscope and put it right on his chest, and he fell asleep. He fell asleep holding the hemostat with my stethoscope on his chest. I remember his son was with him. The patient was right at the end of his life.

Hours later, when I was up at the desk, his son came up to me and said, "These belong to you." I asked him how his father was doing. The son told me his father had died but my letting him hold the hemostat meant an awful lot to him. The son said to me, "Did you know he was a doctor?"

I did not know that. It turned out the family were all doctors. What meaning that must have had for him, to be able to hold that hemostat! The son told me his dad died peacefully.

Gail's experience with her patient and his family showed that even in the short-term interventions that occur with trauma cases, a patient's care could—and should—extend beyond the physical assessment. Though medical intervention failed to save him, Gail's efforts to treat the whole person allowed him to achieve a sense of peace and satisfaction…and a good death.

As Gail continued her work in the emergency department, she began to realize that although there was satisfaction in swift responses and mission accomplished, these were extremely small stages in the recovery of a whole human person:

> In the trauma section we medically stabilized the patient, and they moved to another unit. Some went to the operating room or to a step-down unit. But then another person who arrived would replace them. It was nonstop. In the back of your mind at the end of the day you were so exhausted, and you didn't have time to ask or to find out the outcomes of the patients you had taken care of.
>
> That was a big loss for me, never having a follow-up on how they did afterwards. I thought of that many times because we took care of so many bad gunshot wounds and motor vehicle accidents. *What kinds of outcomes will be possible after such horrible injuries? Was I doing this all wrong? Will the care we gave make a difference?*

Gail wanted to continue utilizing the high-level technical skills she had, but she also wanted to stay with patients, build relationships, and become a part of the care that took place beyond their initial trauma treatment.

Eventually, she returned to Michigan and continued working in the ER. There were many times she was asked to float to the understaffed intensive care areas and she did it willingly. Gail liked the type of nursing she witnessed in the intensive care units. It still required high-tech nursing skills, but it allowed her to spend more time with patients and their families. And it offered her a chance to witness outcomes.

Communication and connections in critical care units

Gail's nursing skills continued to grow as she worked with acutely ill patients in the CCU. Unlike in the ER, in the CCU her interactions with patients' families became routine. As her experience grew, she honed a crucial skill for critical care nurses:

the ability to have empathetic, supportive conversations with patients and family members.

Gail's empathy for CCU families inspired her to campaign for major changes to hospital policy. When Gail approached the hospital's chief nursing officer to advocate for a self-governance model for nurses in the CCU, she succeeded in extending visiting hours. Lengthening the amount of time family members could spend with their critically ill loved one allowed them to become more attuned to their health status. If a patient was deteriorating, the family was less apt to be surprised at an unfavorable turn of events. Just knowing they would be able to spend more time with their loved one decreased family members' anxiety. The new policy benefited the patients as well through increased communication and decreased stress.

It was the beginning of a family-centered approach, but a truly family-centered approach involved much more than expanded visiting hours. Critical care nurses must be able to connect with patients and their families. They must be comfortable discussing emotionally charged topics and delivering medically complex information. Whether it is good news or unwelcome news, whether it involves test results, lab values, or medication, critical care nurses must be able to deliver information to patients and families effectively.

Highly regarded for her ability to connect with people, Gail believes that effective communication in nursing comes not only from knowledge, competence, and objectivity—it also takes practice. She believes that "right out of the gate, you've got to get experience, which is the first step."

In critical care units, good news is always welcomed, and Gail has plenty of good news stories of patients' recoveries in the CCU. She recalls severe cases of pneumonia requiring full ventilator support that were successfully treated with rest and antibiotics, their patients ultimately discharged to return to normal life. There was also good news closer to home after a CCU nurse who had worked alongside Gail for many years developed a blockage of a major artery. This condition is known as "the widowmaker" because it is so deadly. After being emergently admitted, she was treated in the CCU by her own colleagues. A wife and mother with young children, she knew how life-threatening her situation was and she was acutely aware how different it felt to be on the receiving end of the care she had provided for others. Fortunately, she recovered and was able to return to work.

The attention and care Gail offered to patients and their families helped produce these positive moments in the CCU. One family desperately wanted to have a patient baptized. Because the patient was a Baptist, the baptism required a full-body immersion into water. Incredibly, Gail found a tub, obtained permission, and with the help of nursing aides, she made it happen. The family sang as the staff lifted the patient and submerged her into the water. After the baptism, the patient improved and was discharged in a matter of days.

It is wonderful when nurses can share experiences like these with patients and their families, but critical care nursing also requires nurses to deliver unwelcome news about end-of-life diagnoses and treatment failures with no hope of recovery. These conversations take special skills. In these scenarios, Gail found that giving too much information at once or using the typical medical jargon only confused families:

> I learned it is best to give some information and have them repeat it, asking, "What do you think I just said?" That way I would know if we were on the same page and if they understood before going further.

Beyond delivering the medical information, addressing the emotional aspects of these situations can be challenging for healthcare providers. To connect with others during the difficult conversations when treatment is failing, Gail advises:

> The second step is being comfortable talking about one's mortality. How do you best get to that topic and keep somebody listening? So often families will get quite defensive when you talk about anything related to death and dying, but that information—"the patient is dying"—is what needs to be conveyed and understood.
>
> These sorts of conversations were difficult for all healthcare providers. Some have become good at it. Dr. Haydon and I worked together as a team doing this. He would do the medical diagnosis/prognosis, and then I would do the nursing part and follow up with the discussion of the potential quality of life issues. So, Paul and I developed, I think, this really powerful way of helping people understand that there was a shift away from the possibility of recovery.

Dr. Paul Haydon has been working in critical care units for over four decades. His love of medicine started early in his primary education when he realized, "god, I love biochemistry, I love physiology, and I think I could be good at this."

And he was good at it. He was a lead intensivist in the ICU and CCU and taught rotating residents in these settings. He also co-led the hospital's first ethics committee. Standing over 6'4", with broad shoulders and piercing blue eyes, he made an imposing figure as he walked through the units with his white lab coat billowing behind him. His physical presence alone generated acknowledgement. But, as Gail discovered, his knowledge and experience in critical care were the true sources of the respect he earned from peers, patients, and healthcare teams.

Dr. Haydon made it a point to address quality-of-life issues with patients and their families in critical care units. His experiences gave him insight into the physician's role in communicating the benefits and burdens of continued treatment as it relates to a patient's wishes:

> I think everyone dreads being incapacitated to some degree. Everybody has a point, based on their own wishes or quality of life, [when] they would say "this is acceptable" or "this is unacceptable."

> That is where I think the health provider has to step up and promise that, to the best of their ability to predict a [patient's] outcome,…that "this is where we are on that [potential quality of life] value line," if you will.

Gail also needed to manage CCU patients' expectations about quality of life. She learned through experience that a reliable way to understand a patient's expectations was to ask them directly about their wishes for a treatment's outcome:

> I would often use the phrase, "What are you hoping for, in terms of your recovery?" A wealth of information can come from that simple question. But if what they are wishing for is not even possible, the doctors needed to know this and convey that it was not attainable.

Unfortunately, these questions cannot be asked of patients who, due to the severity of their illness, are not able to respond. Instead, nurses must direct their questions to family members or designated surrogates, who then carry the responsibility of decision-making. In those cases, Gail would also try the "What if" approach:

> The easiest way to help people think through decisions that must be made for others is to ask them to imagine if this situation was happening to them. I would ask them, "What if you were unable to recognize your family

members, and you were just lying there unconscious and could not recognize or could not hear? What if you were on machines but not able to understand anybody? How would you feel about that? Would that be [good] quality of life for you? Or, if your loved one were looking down on what was happening right now, what do you think they would tell you to do? Would your loved one say it was [good] quality of life for them?"

The "What if" question was not about presenting every possible medical scenario to the patient, like, "What if you need blood, or what if you need to be under anesthesia for a procedure?" It is about the bigger picture, like, "What if the treatment gets you nowhere?"

This powerful question would sometimes evoke unpredictable replies. There were cases in which the burdens of treatment were so immense that the family, or the patients themselves, would respond, "It is time to stop."

But there were also patients who took a different perspective on the "What if" question, like the young mother of three small children who had end-stage ovarian cancer. She wanted every possible treatment, even up to her last breath. Her response to "What if" was driven by another profound question: "How could I say yes to abandoning my children?"

And so, Gail learned that asking the "What if" question also required a willingness to understand all the responses it evoked.

Family Matters Support Service: A new way of delivering care

Gail's use of empathic listening and clarifying questions became standard in her work with patients and families. These communication skills also became the standard she expected from her staff in the Family Matters Support Service (FMSS) Department.

FMSS was originally the "Family Matters in Critical Care" project, which began at Oakwood Hospital in the early 1990s. Gail and fellow CCU nurse Chris Westphal, MSN, RN, worked together with Dr. Haydon and Linda Barbret, RN, to translate their passion for family-centered care into a series of concrete changes that would improve the quality of care in the CCU. These changes were based on empirical evidence that indicated that the needs of the families of seriously ill patients were not being met (Barbret et al., 1997).

Initially, the project focused on informational resources, such as booklets and posters for the waiting area in the CCU, along with programs to educate staff on how to better support family-centered care. It was financially underwritten by three annual community fundraising events, and, as time went on, it gained the strong support of local hospital leaders and was integrated into three other Detroit metro-area hospitals.

Gail expanded the project by advocating for administrative support to create and coordinate quality improvement projects and small research studies, which provided evidence of its positive outcomes. Eventually, when she observed that more and more ethics consults were requested due to family dissatisfaction and distress, she broadened her advocacy for family-centered care to include "proactive ethics." In her doctoral thesis, Gail argued for proactive interventions that would mitigate potential ethical issues by providing better family support. Her work formed the basis of a subsequent white paper that recommended the development of formal organizations to manage these needs.

Family Matters Support Service became one of these organizations. Founded at Oakwood Hospital in 1998 with Gail and Chris as its dedicated staff, its purpose was to facilitate family education and communication. It combined educational support, spiritual support, and communication and coordination across all hospital disciplines. Eventually, FMSS was implemented system-wide.

The department's name was Dr. Haydon's idea. "Family Matters Support Service" captures what is essential to every patient's care: communication and family. Chris described how the service would integrate families into critical care: "Our intent was for education and support of families who were experiencing the critical illness of a loved one. It quickly moved toward supporting them in making tough decisions."

In order to fulfill its mission of improving communication among healthcare providers and family members, FMSS allowed Gail and her staff to stay with assigned patients throughout their hospital stay, both to learn what was important to them and to get to know them as a part of a family unit. FMSS staff were charged with clearly communicating to patients and families the information they needed to make decisions for their treatment.

Don Johnson, RN, an FMSS nurse, would tell patients and their families to think of him as the *family's* nurse, someone who would be a liaison and help them with the complicated lingo and complexities of hospitalization. His role was to be a constant they could depend on, to help them find answers to their questions, and to explain things in terms they could understand.

A patient might begin receiving FMSS support in a critical care unit or on a general medical floor. No matter where a patient's connection with FMSS began, they would receive support through the resolution of their medical issue. Sometimes the staff member's relationship with the patient would end with their discharge home or to a rehab facility. But there were many times it would end with the patient's death in the hospital. It was not uncommon for family members and Gail to stand side-by-side during a patient's last moments. FMSS staff often became a part of an end-of-life journey.

FMSS allowed Gail to experience aspects of patient care that she felt were missing in the ER and CCU:

> I finally found closure with the Family Matters Service. With trauma, I never had the closure because I never knew what happened to the patients beyond the trauma area. Family Matters brought a lot of closure to all my experiences over the years. That was a really positive thing for me, a very helpful thing for me…It gave meaning to me.

FMSS also recognized that family, and the need for family support, extended beyond just our human connections. One of the unique ways Family Matters staff made a difference was to develop a program for visits from patients' own pets. It was called Pet Affection Wins Smiles (PAWS). Gail recalls how the pet therapy protocol was established:

> There was a 95-year-old lady that was dying. She wasn't conversational, but she would yell out, "Zoe! Where is Zoe? I just must see Zoe."

> When a friend came to visit her, I asked who Zoe was and found out it was her dog. She was a big white husky. I made two calls to administrators and told them I would make sure that the safety issues were addressed.

> I brought Zoe in through the ER and thank heavens she was well-behaved. I brought her up to the patient, and the dog immediately jumped right up on the bed and on her chest. The patient had no teeth. She was 95 and practically bald. Zoe placed her paws right by her neck and gave her a big kiss. I still have a picture of that. Then she just put her head on the patient's shoulder and closed her eyes. It was just beautiful. We just kept things quiet and let them be alone. Zoe stayed about a half hour, and then I took her back down to her caregiver, who was waiting in the ER. By the time I got back up to see the patient, she had passed. She had a smile on her face.

That was when the pet therapy program really started, which evolved into a big project. We had scarves for the pets to wear to identify them as a *Special Visitor*. Dogs and cats came to visit. We had no incidents other than heartwarming ones. For many patients and pets, it was their last time together.

Gail also discovered other profound ways that the staff could express care to patients. Family Matters Support Service started delivering "love blankets," or lap covers knitted or sewn by volunteers.

The love blanket idea originated when Gail decided to give a colorful scarf to a young mother who was dying. It was for the benefit of the patient's daughter, who Gail was worried about. Gail had the girl place it on her mother as a sort of hug to wrap around her and keep her safe. The next day when Gail was walking down the hall, she saw the young girl leaving the room with the scarf around her own neck. Her mother had died. "I will always keep this," the daughter told her.

Draping the handmade blanket across the stark white hospital spread often became a special moment. It seemed that when a love blanket was given to a patient, something magical happened, something beyond the scope of traditional medicine: the love blanket coincidentally would be the patient's favorite color, or it would draw family members closer to the bedside to finally touch the patient. There were countless love blanket stories. It never failed that if the patient was responsive, they were delighted and moved to receive this unexpected gift. Their family members were just as grateful and surprised. Gail remembers:

> I went to see a patient who was terminally ill. His wife of 50 plus years was at his bedside, as well as his adult children. I had just returned from picking up several bags of love blankets, made of cut-and-tied fleece and donated from an out-of-area high school. Our blanket supply in

Family Matters was low, and so I was happy to take one out of this new supply to give him. When I unfolded the blanket and placed it on him, I explained that it was a gift, that sometimes something soft and colorful brought comfort that words could not. When I mentioned what high school donated it, his wife started crying. "We were both students there," she said. "That is where we met and fell in love."

Even though they may be small, connections such as these illustrate the sacredness of the end-of-life space and show how closing the circle does not just finish it, it makes it whole. Over time, Family Matters Support Service interventions evolved into a holistic approach that honored patient experiences, values, spirituality, family relationships, and cultural norms. They assisted patients in tying up loose ends, expressing loss or grief, and accepting outcomes. By meeting these needs at whatever level they are attainable, FMSS staff contributed to what Gail refers to as a good death.

Another element of a good death was highlighted by the case of "Thomas." Gail's account of his passing reveals the significance of self-determination in closing one's circle:

> There was a patient I will call "Thomas" who was 86 years old and in the cardiac care unit. He was receiving the most supportive care available because of a recent heart attack. Already on dialysis for several years from kidney disease, he was in a very weakened state. But his mind was clear. Hooked to monitors and intravenous tubing, he looked dwarfed in a room containing a sea of technology.
>
> As head nurse of CCU, I was present for most of the conversations that occurred between Thomas and the physicians. Every day we touched base, and I listened to his questions and concerns. I believe this is truly the most critical aspect of care in the aftermath of serious illness: the

ability to communicate and to make decisions based on a quality of life that is acceptable to you. Thomas had decided that he did not want to be resuscitated if his heart stopped.

It was 5 a.m. when Thomas asked if I would arrange for his family to come in later that day. "It is not an emergency. I just want to talk to them," he said. It took a couple of hours for everyone to get there. I could see the family in Thomas's room through a large observation window. They took turns shifting from the bedside to the window to any vacant space. They exchanged places for hand holding, and saying "I love you." When the entire family was present, as well as the hospital's priest, I was asked to join them around the bed. Glancing from face to face I could see an array of emotions.

Despite the equipment that beeped and flashed, the wires and tubes that draped from poles and became tethers confounding embraces, it was Thomas who took command of the hospital room. One by one, he addressed each person. One by one, he thanked them, told them he loved them, and provided a personal comment based on their importance to him and his life. He then thanked me and my staff for the care he had received. He said he was tired and then slowly closed his eyes.

As a cardiac nurse you are trained to be ever-watchful of the patient's heart monitor, and so my glance from Thomas's face to the monitor above his bed was second nature. Even though I had seen many unexplainable and spiritual occurrences in my career, I was amazed to see the immediacy in which the peaks and valleys that indicate heart activity become a smooth, still line. While family was still gathered around him, Thomas had died. He had included loved ones in his death and given them permission to be as much a part of his life's ending as they had been throughout it. In a profoundly intimate and inclusive way, Thomas had closed his circle.

The story about Thomas is true but, sadly, uncommon. Rather than calm, deliberate decisions and communication, it is more likely that breathing machines, powerful medications, deteriorating body systems, and unconscious patients result in turmoil for the family members faced with medical decision-making.

The more common story is one in which the critically ill person had never shared what sort of existence would be acceptable and unacceptable. It is a story in which family members either shun or overstep their roles in medical decision-making—and of how the family unit fractures under the strain of loss and the guilt and fear of making a wrong decision. Gail relates how FMSS worked to help patients and families facing end-of-life challenges:

> Our goal in Family Matters was to help the family and help the patient and to make sure they had adequate communication and all the facts they needed to make a good decision. There were many times families would come in, and they were so distraught about what they would see—all the IVs, ventilators, machines. They were so overcome with grief and not really able at that time to process medical information.
>
> It was the environment that the patient and family were in that always made it a double-edged sword. You had to not only deal with the patient and the doctors but now the whole family. Some of them might not even agree with each other. So, it is really a complex balancing and juggling ordeal. Sometimes trying to keep everybody on the same page almost takes a miracle in some cases.

A grassroots foundation for clinical ethics

While Gail and the FMSS staff helped many patients and families, not every FMSS case could be resolved through increased communication and family support. Increasingly complex critical illnesses and the advancement of medical technology have challenged the healthcare system, complicating the determinations of medical decision-makers, the use of scarce resources, and the physician's professional assessment of whether continued treatment could even result in a beneficial outcome.

Cases that involved these challenges sometimes required an ethics consultation. When there was a concern that ethical principles were being compromised, an ethics consult identified what ethical principle was being tested, analyzed the ramifications, and provided a recommendation for resolution. Sometimes additional scrutiny of ethical standards was required, conducted by selected members from the ethics committee. Gail and Dr. Haydon began the first multidisciplinary ethics committee at Oakwood when Gail was still the head nurse in the CCU. Eventually Gail, who continued her education while working full time, earned a PhD in Interdisciplinary Studies with a focus on ethics and end-of-life care.

Dr. Haydon recalls the early stage of the clinical ethics committee:

> We were not educated in terms of ethical reasoning or how to process the whole thing. It started out as trying to do the right thing for the population that we were serving. But quickly it became issues of how do [the family members] accept or not accept death, and under what context do they accept death? It just snowballed.

> And of course, you would have the reproductive people involved, and what were we doing with our embryos? So, suddenly, all these medical issues popped up. Based on those who were the experts and those who were in the trenches, we were interested in getting more formalized and asking the question: "Am I doing it the right way?"

> I think we started out more of a grassroots group of people at [Oakwood Hospital and Medical Center] that just shared the same vision of, boy, how do we sort out the

right way to do some of this in terms of the delivery of health care? Then we finally sat down, and we realized that you cannot be inbred. We needed a professional ethicist.

Gail worked with Dr. Haydon to expand the committee to a team of people who were resolute in their commitment to upholding ethical principles in the clinical setting:

> It changed from being all physicians to a multidisciplinary team. The committee included nurses, social workers, Father Rich, lawyers, and others. We formed this multidisciplinary group, and it was wonderful. It was the place where you could talk about these tough cases with seemingly no real right or wrong answers. That is how it all started, and it just grew from there.

> Then people like Nursing Administrator Barb Hertzler, along with other administrators, financially supported and created the first position in clinical ethics and appointed me as the Director of the Clinical Ethics Consultation Service. It was a paid position thanks to Barb's support, and it allowed me to step away from CCU and have Family Matters as well as the clinical ethics service become my sole focus.

But the committee still needed a seasoned professional to guide and educate them. Leonard Weber, PhD, was asked to participate as the hospital's medical ethicist. Dr. Weber was a respected ethics consultant throughout the Metro Detroit area and a founding member of the Medical Ethics Resource Network of Michigan (MERN). With gray hair and unwavering dark eyes, he gave the impression of a more refined, modern-day Merlin. He mentored, taught, guided, and questioned—not from a book of magic, but based on his 30 years on the faculty of University of Detroit Mercy and the four books and over 90 articles that he published during his career. With a broad range of experience under his belt, he brought the expertise needed to whip a grassroots effort into shape.

Ethical issues can arise because of differences between a patient and a family member, among family members, between a family and a medical team, or between hospital regulations and a person's right to refuse treatment. Dr. Weber made sure discussions were conducted within the framework of ethical reasoning, educated the staff on the application of medical ethics in the clinical setting, and provided oversight for the recommendations the ethics committee was asked to make. He explained:

> The whole concept of medical ethics is based on the idea that we need to bring some ethical organization, ethical perspectives, to bear on these hard medical decisions. As soon as you bring in ethicists, you have people who are trying to sort through what kind of criteria you use, and that is what the ethical principles are, decision-making criteria.

Dr. Weber taught Gail and her team how a person's perspective could influence their goals. They also learned that a patient's goals can be a pivotal part of their treatment decisions.

One such case involved "Alice," an African American woman in her late seventies who had been admitted for aspiration pneumonia, a condition that occurs when the swallowing muscles become weak. Instead of fluid or food going to the stomach, it gets diverted into the lungs. Untreated pneumonia can be life threatening and requires medical treatment. Serious cases require hospitalization and sometimes the temporary use of a breathing machine.

After two previous admissions for the same condition, the attending physician recommended a permanent feeding tube for Alice based on the likelihood of continued aspiration, which put her life at risk. This would mean that all her nourishment would be liquid and delivered by a tube placed directly through her abdominal wall and into the stomach. She would no longer eat or drink normally. The attending physician believed it was his professional obligation to require that the feeding tube be inserted before the patient was discharged home.

Alice was living independently at the time and had family members close by who were attentive to her. She was her own decision-maker and was mentally competent. She also understood the concerns of the medical team and the reasons they wanted to put the tube directly into her stomach. But she absolutely refused to have the feeding tube inserted, explaining that eating and tasting food was part of what made life meaningful for her. Alice would not consent to the medical advice, and the physician did not want to authorize her discharge.

After confirming that Alice had a full understanding of her condition and the risks to herself, the ethics consultation team determined that she had the right to "informed refusal" of the feeding tube placement. The ethics team also recommended that she and her family meet with the hospital's nutritionist to become educated on how to swallow with less risk, the foods that would be a safer option, and the signs that indicated she had aspirated.

In Alice's case, the clinical ethics committee assisted the healthcare team by recommending that this course of action was the correct one, despite their misgivings. The ethics team's presence at Oakwood became instrumental in determining how to "sort out the right way to do things" in the ethical delivery of healthcare.

Good policy and advance directives

Although every ethics case is different, the complicated cases that arose in Gail's career influenced her dedication to create strong policy. She recognized the importance of setting standards of care that are legally sound, ethical, and consistently applied to all patients. She helped develop and update policies about code status, advance directives, withholding and withdrawing treatment, brain death, and informed consent, among others. The policies helped to ensure that even when opinions differed, all patients would benefit from consistent standards and thoughtful, deliberate application of principles and policy.

This conviction also drove Gail, Chris Westphal, and a team of like-minded peers to draw from their FMSS experience and the work of Linda and Ezekiel Emanuel (1989), both renowned physicians and bioethicists, to produce an award-winning advance directive document, aptly named *My Voice - My Choice*. This document encouraged conversation prior to critical circumstances and named a medical decision-making spokesperson chosen by the patient. As a legally binding document, it met the statutory requirements for advance directives and power of attorney for healthcare. However, it differed from other advance directives because it included exercises to facilitate discussions and clarify values related to serious illness and end-of-life care. It was distributed to and completed by thousands of patients, both within the hospital setting and in the community. It was eventually printed in Spanish and Arabic.

Gail's work to produce, promote, and educate people about advance directives is a culmination of the many lessons she learned during her career. One could say that it is this lesson—to complete an advance directive—that Gail hoped everyone would learn. She believed that openly talking about and documenting one's end-of-life wishes could make the difference between a good, a bad, or even an ugly death.

Gail's personal and professional journey led to important advances in patients' right to self-determination and the consistent application of ethical standards to all patients in any circumstance. In addition to learning from her own experiences, she sought out and united with others who had the courage to take on these complex and often emotionally challenging issues.

The synergy, passion, and dedication among Gail, Dr. Haydon, Dr. Weber, and their colleagues not only gave rise to Oakwood Hospital's first advance directive document, it also resulted in a wealth of other important insights about end-of-life care. The lessons they learned about closing the circle are shared in the chapters that follow.

Join our Circle

Just as Gail joined together with her colleagues to provide better end-of-life care for patients and their families, we invite you to join us in discussing the lessons they learned from their experiences.

The chapters that follow each present a different dimension of closing the circle. At the end of each chapter, we've included questions designed to help you reflect on the chapter's subject matter and explore your own experiences and insights.

In this chapter, we followed Gail on her personal and professional journey.

- Where are you on your planned trajectory of your healthcare career?

- What experiences have changed the course of your career or your mindset for how you practice?

- Are there lessons that you have learned that would be valuable to share with others?

Chapter 2

Trust, Truth, and Informed Consent: The Healthcare Provider's Impact on Medical Decision-Making

From the first time a person walks into your office, they are your patient; you have a contract with them. This is the principle of fidelity: an obligation to do the best you can for them. It also means telling them the truth. I can't treat them without telling them what I am treating them for, even when other family members want to shield them from bad news. Patients have faith in our relationship. To not tell the truth would be to lie, and I can't do that. But I also tell my patients if you ever find a doctor that tells you they know everything, run like hell.

—George Hnatiuk, MD

In our work with Gail and Family Matters, we saw firsthand how important it is for patients to trust their healthcare providers, particularly when they are facing difficult or complicated medical decisions. Gail built trust with patients and families through honesty and clear communication. She was far ahead of her time in making medical information readily available to them. She would bring a chart into the patient's room or to a family meeting and methodically explain the test results and consultation notes, checking in with them frequently

to make sure they understood what she was saying.

Gaining patients' trust is essential for all healthcare providers, but it isn't always easy. In this chapter, we share the perspectives of doctors and other healthcare providers we've worked with who depended on their patients' trust to provide ethical and effective care, and their thoughts on how to establish that trust.

When faced with a serious illness, patients and their family members should have an accurate understanding of the illness, its potential treatments, and those treatments' probability of success before they are asked to make any decisions. However, sometimes simply presenting the information is not enough: patients and family members must believe that the information is coming from a trustworthy source.

Trust: The healthcare provider's perspective

Gail's colleague George Hnatiuk, MD, had a primary care practice in internal medicine and a subspecialty in hematology. He had a remarkable ability to connect to the patients and families in his practice, which spanned over 40 years. Four of his patients were over 100 years old when he retired, and he had cared for them since they were in their 60s. His approachable demeanor and compassionate honesty earned him both his peers' and his patients' trust. Dr. Hnatiuk described how he built trust between himself and his patients, and how it impacted his work:

> You develop a relationship with patients, and they become part of my family, and I became part of their family. I knew about them, their parents, their children, and grandchildren. If they know you and they know you are doing everything you can for them, and that you have always been there for them when they need you, it makes a difference. They accepted what I told them needed to be done. That helps build that trust, and I think that trust is

important to go on with the next step. I think it is very, very important.

Establishing trust with patients, especially before their health starts to decline, provides a sense of security for them and their families, which is particularly important if the patient is faced with a serious or complicated illness.

Dr. Haydon believes that primary care physicians are often in the best position to establish trust with their patients due to the close relationship they can develop with them:

> I feel strongly that the healthcare delivery system must be built on the primary care doctor. And to that end, they have the relationship, the knowledge, and the experience. When I have a primary care doctor who knows these people, again, it is so much easier.

> I have seen some very good primary physicians tell the patient, "I've spoken to the heart specialist," or "I've spoken to the stomach specialist, and here's what they are recommending."

> If the patient's relationship with their primary is solid, it works. But if a relationship has not been established, then they do not trust what is being relayed to them, and they want to hear it directly from the specialist. And even then, they may not trust what the specialist says and will ask, "What did the MRI show?"

With the advent of easy access to medical information on the internet, Dr. Haydon found that some patients and family members attempt to interpret medical values and information themselves, rather than trust in a physician's medical experience and opinion:

> It is quite simple. [As a specialist] either I am going to be asked my opinion of what the future holds, with an understanding it is not 100% predictable, or somebody will

ask me what a test result is. If you ask me what I think, it is going to be more valuable. If you ask me what the complete blood count was or the MRI was, like most people do because they do not trust my opinion, you are back to square one…So there needs to be an element of trust.

When a patient's relationship with a physician is built on trust, the patient and family are more likely to rely on the physician's expert interpretation, rather than trying to decipher hourly changes in blood chemistry or fluctuating vital signs themselves. Their ability to trust their physician can alleviate unnecessary stress during a difficult time. In today's world of complex and abundant treatment options, relying on a physician's expertise may also reduce the patient's emotional distress about which choices to make.

But even when there is a trusting relationship with the healthcare provider, unanticipated outcomes can throw the family into disarray. As a palliative care nurse practitioner, Chris Westphal observed how new advanced treatment options can also make it more difficult for families to recognize the point when a treatment will no longer return a patient to health or be in the patient's best interest:

> When I first started my nursing career, patients were intubated for surgery, and post-op they were extubated. That was that. There were no long-term ventilators, no tracheostomies or long-term care facilities. There were not places people went to live on life support.

With the life-sustaining technologies that now exist, a patient may end up in a circumstance their family members never imagined. For example, a medical intervention may have allowed a patient to survive a crisis, but then the patient may become dependent on ventilator support for the rest of their life. A patient with kidney disease might require lifelong dialysis, or placement in an extended care facility for specialized nursing care. Although life-sustaining resources are now much more sophisticated than they were in the past, sometimes they are still not enough. Dr. Hnatiuk described his experience with family members who were not prepared to accept that despite the available medical treatment, their loved one was not going to get better:

> I think they are angry. They do not believe you. They think there is always something that can be done and there is always someone out there that can help them, so they want to be referred to a doctor they heard about. Or they saw one specialist and say, "Well, we heard there was another one and wanted her." Or they want to go to Mayo Clinic. In my experience it is mostly families this happens with. I think the patients, as a rule, probably realize they are reaching the end zone. But families do not want to let go sometimes.

Sudden critical illness can elicit difficult emotions and often prompt the patient's or family's request to "do everything," including pursuing even the most invasive treatments with a low probability of success. This knee-jerk response can stem from emotions that hinder the ability to absorb and accept vital information, such as the fact that the patient is dying. As ethicist Paul Reitemeier, PhD, said, "As soon as fear is elicited—like hearing, 'You have cancer'— nothing else can be heard that day."

This sort of emotional upheaval is intensified if there is a lack of trust between the patient and the healthcare team. But how can this trust be established, especially in a world of changing providers and multiple consultants?

Gail discovered in her experience as a nurse, establishing trust begins with effective truth-telling. Healthcare providers must be straightforward about what a treatment can and cannot do, and deliver that information in understandable terms.

Truth-telling with clarity and compassion

When a patient or their family or spokesperson is asked to consent to a treatment, it is important for them to understand not only what they are consenting to, but also what the expected outcomes could be.

Here are some examples of how a healthcare provider might explain a treatment's expected outcomes to the patient and family:

> "Once we start dialysis, we may have to continue it for the rest of Ruby's life."

> "There are side effects that can occur when chemotherapy is introduced. We can help to minimize them, but they can be challenging. Here are some of the best-case and worst-case scenarios."

> "Because you have end-stage lung disease, it is very likely that if you are put on the ventilator you may not be able to survive without it. This would mean having a permanent breathing tube and the need for 24-hour care providers."

For the healthcare provider, truth-telling is the act of empathetically presenting the facts even when they will disrupt a patient's life. It requires conveying unwelcome news in understandable terms with consideration for how it will impact the patient and their loved ones.

Dr. Reitemeier believes truth-telling is one of the key principles in medical decision-making and the most important of ethical principles in healthcare. He states, "If you start with truth, you rarely get into trouble. If you don't start with the truth, you almost always get into trouble."

Dr. Reitemeier has over 30 years' experience in ethics. His education started when medical ethics was just beginning to develop in academia. The field was so new that he had to design his own medical ethics course for his master's degree. He could cite chapter and verse in most ethics tomes. While he advocates truth-telling, he also acknowledges that healthcare providers may be hesitant to deliver unwelcome news, and that patients may give the impression that they don't want to hear it. To address this challenge, he recommends delivering difficult information in terms that are understandable and humanistic:

> You can ease people into accepting very difficult unwanted truths if it is compassionately delivered—and, if it is delivered at the speed the heart can absorb. We give it at the speed we think their brain can take. But it is the heart that takes time.
>
> Those with resistance to hearing the truth? It's not that they don't want to know. They desperately want to know. They just don't want it to be true.

For healthcare providers, medical truth-telling can sometimes feel like walking a tightrope. While it is essential to gently deliver the facts, it's also important not to overwhelm the patient with information while they are processing difficult news. Dr. Reitemeier cites advice offered by Oliver Wendel Holmes, Sr., a writer, doctor, and educator who lived in the horse-and-buggy days of the late 1800s: "Your patient has no more right to all the truth you know than he has to all the medicine in your saddlebag…He should only get just so much as is good for him" (Holmes, 1892, p. 388).

Holmes knew it is not the responsibility of the patient or their decision-maker to sort through all the medical information, or to determine the course of treatment. Instead, they must trust their physician to do so.

Dr. Reitemeier had his own experience with truth-telling with his mother at the end of her life. When she asked him whether she was dying, he relied on the trust between them to respond to her question in a compassionate way that wouldn't overwhelm or frighten her:

> I knew the answer, and I kind of hedged because I also knew if I told her the truth that she could come back with a negative, sort of mom-ish retort like, "What the hell do you know?"
>
> I said to her, "Only the good lord knows."
>
> And she said, "Well, then ask him!"
>
> As soon as she said that the room broke into laughter, and she did too. That was the release—the emotional cathartic release that was needed—and she had her answer.

Each relationship between a healthcare provider and a patient and family is different. Some may have met only recently, while others may have built a relationship up over decades. While a physician or other provider may need to adjust their approach accordingly, patients should always hear the comprehensive truth delivered with clarity and compassion.

The hidden trust of informed consent

The ethical principle of informed consent requires that medical decision-making should only take place after a patient or caregiver has a full understanding of the treatment options and their possible outcomes. Dr. Weber prefers to call this principle "informed decision-making":

> It is common knowledge that one must sign consent for any medical treatment today. In hospitals this is known as an informed consent policy. The two key components to an informed consent are, one, that you are obviously informed and, two, that the person has capacity to consent. In my mind, when you talk about medical decision-making, informed consent is still the primary principle in medical ethics.

Dr. Weber also points out a fundamental difference between the roles of the patient and the physician in informed consent. While the patient is the ultimate decision-maker, the physician is the one who determines the appropriate options, based on their medical knowledge and the current standard of care:

> Informed consent is a responsive role. Informed consent means I consent, or I do not consent. But [the patient] does not initiate what it is [they're] consenting to, because [they] don't have the experience.

The role of a physician is distinct *because* of their level of expertise, which provides a basis for the patient's trust. A patient who is being asked to consent to a treatment must trust that the physician has used their expertise to determine and present the best treatment options.

For some patients and their families, it may be difficult to trust a physician not only because of a lack of personal relationship, but also due to cultural differences, or residual trauma from historical events.

One example of this is the post-WWII discovery of Nazi medical experimentation. Another is the egregious Tuskegee study—a 40-year experiment conducted in the United States on Black males with syphilis that was done without informing the study's subjects or offering them the cure, which was available (Adashi et al., 2018). These extreme examples of medical exploitation and malpractice represent the polar opposite of informed consent and an unforgivable breach of trust between doctor and patient.

As Dr. Weber points out, medical ethics gained greater recognition as a field of study when people began to say, "Wait. You can't do that."

The damage of these events still lingers, but despite these and other challenges, healthcare providers can build trust with patients through effective truth-telling. By communicating clearly and compassionately, physicians and other healthcare providers can help patients understand and accept medical outcomes. Creating relationships that allow patients to put their faith in those that are caring for them is another essential element of helping patients and their loved ones close the circle.

Join our Circle

- Relationships between patients and healthcare providers are more effective if they are based on trust. **How do you begin to establish trust with a new patient?**

- Dr. Haydon found that it was easier to provide good care when patients trusted his medical expertise, rather than trying to interpret their own medical tests and values. **Have you worked with patients or families who have tried to research and interpret complicated test results and medical data themselves? How did you respond?**

- Dr. Reitemeier said, "You can ease people into accepting very difficult unwanted truths if it is compassionately delivered—and, if it is delivered at the speed the heart can absorb." **What techniques do you use to deliver difficult information in understandable terms and in a compassionate way?**

- When Dr. Reitemeier had to deliver difficult medical news to his mother, he adapted his form of medical truth-telling to suit their relationship. **What are some ways that you can adapt your communication style to better connect with a patient or a family?**

Chapter 3

Unpacking Autonomy: The Family's Role in Medical Decision-Making

When we seek for connection, we restore the world
to wholeness. Our seemingly separate lives become
meaningful as we discover how truly necessary we are to
each other.

—Margaret Wheatley

Every healthcare provider begins their work in the field expecting to spend a good deal of time with patients, but some don't realize how often they will be interacting with patients' families. Patients' families can play an enormous role in medical decision-making, either directly or indirectly.

When Gail and Chris began Family Matters its mission was not just a good idea—it was a necessity. They not only offered additional support to families in and out of the hospital setting, they also assisted the healthcare team in integrating the family into the patient's care. In this chapter, we hope to assist you by offering our colleagues' insights on how to work with families, especially during stressful, high-stakes situations and end-of-life care.

The importance of family

Even before a child can speak or think rationally, their world is already being formed by nuances of cultural and personal meaning supplied by their primary caregivers. The families we are raised in are part of a cultural framework that consists of norms, of "shoulds" and "shouldn'ts," passed along from generation to generation. In its earliest days, a child's family creates its reality.

And despite all the upheavals in family relationships that can occur over a lifetime, family often continues to affect our actions in our adulthood. Family values serve as a measuring stick to evaluate the world and its priorities, a foundational influence on our perspective and decisions. Family matters.

The impact of family on a patient's care needs to be acknowledged and managed by all healthcare providers because, in most cases, families are a constant presence. The family's activities in a hospital setting may range from a friendly bedside visit during a patient's uneventful recovery to a frantic assembly following an emergency phone call when a loved one is in medical distress. Family may be included in meetings with physicians to help provide patient support, and in many cases family members must take on the role of decision-maker.

Gail, Chris, and Dr. Haydon recognized the influence of family in their everyday experiences working in critical care. Dr. Haydon suggested the name "Family Matters" for the new support department Gail and Chris wanted to form because he believed the patient's family needed to be a more prominent consideration as a part of patient care. Chris explained:

> We started Family Matters in the early 1990s under the umbrella of the clinical ethics department. Our Family Matters model was based on data that suggested that cases were being brought to clinical ethics not because

of medical issues but because of communication issues. At that time, the recommendation was to have this new avenue to address any communication issues first, and if it truly was an ethical dilemma, then it became a clinical ethics consult.

The communication issues Gail and Chris were seeing grew out of the challenges healthcare providers faced when integrating families into the patient's care. Providers often needed to balance patient confidentiality with clear and helpful communication to those family members who are at the patient's bedside. With multiple providers attending to a patient and a rotating cast of family members in and out of the room, it could be difficult to ensure that everyone was accurately informed. The pace at which decisions needed to be made around a patient's treatment could also leave gaps in communicating the plan to family members, causing confusion, anxiety, or anger.

Though the service was created for a specific purpose, Family Matters evolved to have a broader effect on Oakwood Hospital. Although the stories we refer to as Family Matters cases come from Family Matters staff, they involved many other members of the healthcare team, including physicians, social workers, chaplains, and other ancillary staff, all working together. The work and success of the Family Matters service was only possible because of the coordination and support of many people.

The need for a service that supported both patients and their families became even more important as healthcare transformed from a physician-dominated and paternalistic decision-making model, to a model in which the patient was seen as an autonomous decision-maker, and then to a shared decision-making model that involves both the patient and the family.

But what about autonomy?

A shared decision-making model considers the impact and relationship of family and how it influences a patient's decision-making. It does not take away a patient's right to choose. Instead, it recognizes the role that family plays in the decision-making process. According to Chris:

> Family-centered care recognizes that the patient is a part of this family unit, and what happens to the patient affects the family. And what is happening in the family is affecting the patient. So, when we provide care, we cannot assume, "I am only taking care of you. You are my patient." Unfortunately, some of the healthcare providers will say, "I talk to the patient. I do not talk to the family." Well, if you went into the hospital and saw my dad when he was sick, you could talk to him. It would look like he was registering, but he was not.

Here, Chris is referring to when her father, Art Giska, was hospitalized and a cardiologist recommended a pacemaker for his bradycardia (slow heart rate). Because her father wasn't having any concerning symptoms, he initially expressed that he didn't want one. But when he was approached by a cardiology resident at a time when family wasn't with him, Art agreed to the pacemaker. Luckily, during an early morning visit, Chris's husband found out about the plan and prevented the procedure from being done so that another conversation could take place. Chris wasn't trying to prevent her dad from changing his mind. Rather, she just wanted to be confident this was what he wanted. As it turned out, Art hadn't understood and he didn't want the pacemaker. He just needed help sorting his decision out.

In Chris's father's case, and in many others, the patient's family was able to assist with communicating information to a person who was not capable of understanding what was happening, or who was too stressed or ill to be able to retain the medical details that are important for decision-making. This is one major benefit of family participation in patient care.

Despite this and other advantages, some see the idea of family-centered care or "shared decision-making" as potentially in conflict with self-determination and the idea of autonomy. However, Chris agrees with Dr. Weber's belief that making informed decisions requires understanding, and that this often involves the expertise and support of others:

> [Shared decision-making] fosters autonomy because to be autonomous in your decisions, I think you must be informed, educated. I can make an autonomous decision, just a gut reaction, but if I had all the facts would I make that same decision? I think shared decision-making enables the person to get the best information so they can make the best decision for themselves. But they need information. They need the pros and the cons.

In 2011, Ronald Epstein and Richard Street wrote that shared decision-making is an important underlying component for ethical decision-making. It is based on the premise that a patient's right to self-determination can be compromised by high stress and fatigue and that the patient may need help from others to process information. Epstein also argues that autonomy recognizes the value of relationships, and that cooperative decision-making helps to create coherence and meaning.

Family Matters staff member Martha Hnatiuk recalls encountering an easy acceptance of shared decision-making among nursing students:

> When I was teaching a medical ethics class to a group of nurses who were in a BSN completion program, we discussed the idea of shared decision-making. One

Filipino nurse who was in her forties said that, culturally, she would never make a medical decision for herself independently of her family members, and in fact, would expect them to make the decision for her. Others in the class said they would want to be their own decision-maker but that the feedback and support of their family would factor into a decision that they made.

Medical decision-making does not happen in a vacuum. A patient's choice can impact not only their life but also the lives of their loved ones. Patients worry about how their family members may be burdened as they begin to experience diminishing health, complex and ongoing treatments, and increasing dependency. The reliance on loved ones is even stronger when a patient's competency is in question. Shared decision-making reflects how "no man is an island": while patient autonomy is foundational, family participation in patient care can assist with a patient's self-determination, rather than endanger it.

Family Matters and the family

Foster and McLellan (2002) describe families as "relationships marked by dynamic and ethical interconnectedness—past, present and future…that exist among people whose very being has significance for each other" (p. 41).

Their definition acknowledges that identifying family, or "next of kin" as they are often called, is not always straightforward. Some people come from large extended families, or blended families, or families whose members are spread out across states and even different countries. Today when we ask patients about the makeup of their families, the response may not include a spouse or blood relation but rather a person or people they consider to be of primary importance to them. Maybe it is a friend or partner. In one Family Matters case, Gail recalls it was a landlord:

Fred had been taken to the hospital when he was found unresponsive in a local park. After a couple of days in intensive care he was able to answer questions and indicated that he wanted his landlord to be his medical spokesperson if needed. The landlord was asked to come into the hospital and was totally taken aback that Fred wanted him to take on this role. Fred admitted he had relatives, but they were not in his life, and he chose to keep it that way. We helped Fred and his landlord fill out the paperwork to make this decision legally recognized.

There is a new recognition in healthcare that the term *family* means whoever the patient identifies as family when they are asked by healthcare providers. Family Matters did whatever was necessary to support all types of families. Family Matters staff met family members at bedside and in waiting rooms and made both domestic and international phone calls. Communication sometimes involved calls to prison inmates or the use of interpreters, and always required a detailed record of each family member's contact information.

Every day, Family Matters staff did a chart review of the patient's medical status, spoke with the care providers, conducted a bedside visit, and fielded calls from family. According to the model that Gail and Chris pioneered, staff were trained to participate in sensitive discussions with family members that could involve anything from who would be a spokesperson to when to withdraw life support.

Martha Hnatiuk, MA, RN, was a Family Matters staff member for many years. A cheerful, empathetic woman with a warm smile, she began her career as a floor nurse at Oakwood, left to pursue an MA in philosophy, and then taught critical thinking and medical ethics. Martha eventually returned to the clinical setting to take on the role of nurse clinician in the Clinical Ethics Consultation Service and

Family Matters. She described a typical patient consult:

> After a review of the medical record, it was a matter of getting to know this patient and family. I would ask questions to find out what their baseline of information was and how they perceived what was going on. The goal at first was to build a rapport and for me to get a sense of who all the family members were. I also wanted to know about the cognitive, physical, and emotional state of the patient. It was particularly important to find out if the patient had ever written an advance medical directive about their treatment wishes, and if so, if they were still the same wishes, and if the family and physician were aware of them.

She also offered insight about the most effective ways to talk with family members:

> Key factors I learned: Don't rush. Find out each step of the way what the level of understanding was regarding whatever was the medical issue. Provide contact info, and follow up with any calls, and include everyone that you can. Be honest about what you do not know or cannot predict. Be respectful of everyone, and do not take sides even if you have an urge to do so. Show that you care. Maybe this is the most important part. You must be 100 percent there, open.

Reverend Tony Marshall, DMin, who is currently the Clinical Pastoral Education (CPE) Program Manager at the University of Michigan Hospital in Ann Arbor, served as a Spiritual Support Services Chaplain, Director of Spiritual Care, and Coordinator of CPE at Oakwood. He reflected on his work with families and building relationships:

> You come along with families. It is an honor because families welcome us in for the moment. It is really amazing to me how I can walk in a room, and I have never seen

these people before—a mom and dad, or a dad is here on the bed perhaps in the dying process. I can walk in, and that family, for a moment, it is like they bring you in. You become part of their system, become part of their family, and that just blows me away.

This sentiment expressed by Rev. Marshall is a familiar experience for most Family Matters staff. It may happen because serious illness exposes such a vulnerable aspect of being mortal, and when confronting the possibility of the patient's death, the family experiences a deep need to connect with others.

Mary Catherine Wright, MSN, RN, has held many roles in her nursing career, including FMSS clinical nurse specialist. Her very fair skin once earned her the affectionate title of the "whitest white person" when she worked as a parish nurse in an African American church. She also served as a hospice nurse, an administrator for a nursing home, and for many years the only Family Matters nurse in a satellite hospital. A deeply devoted Catholic, her vocabulary could nevertheless be as salty as a sailor, and her entrance into most meetings was accompanied by papers flying and extra bags loaded down with "important stuff." Mary Catherine deeply understood how to connect with and understand patients and their families. She recounted:

> A lot of times in the hospital a patient was so sick that [they couldn't participate and] we had to sit down with the family. You have to develop trust. A person is not going to spill their guts right away. Like Gail would say, "What is common? What do we have in common?"

> When you are dealing with a person at end-of-life you have to include the family. It's not a separate issue. Sometimes the nurses in the unit would be mad at me, claiming the family has no right to make decisions if they

are not the guardians, but you have to consider the family. They are like an appendage of the patient.

Mary Catherine often saw the importance of relationships during a health crisis:

> Some people want to talk. I have had people just talking my ear off. One of my clients in hospice had kind of a negative experience, and I was sent in to do some damage control. When I got there, she told me that all she wanted was for me to get to know her. It was hard because she was my age, and it was tough. I still remember her. I still remember her face and her family. We talked, and then I said that we needed to talk to her husband, and she told me that she could not do it by herself. She was just trying to let go. So, I told her, "I will talk for you." We had the husband sit down, and we talked, and she passed away peacefully. That was a tough case. She just wanted to talk, and she wanted someone to know her and to manage her pain, and I was able to do that.

This profound experience happened repeatedly to Family Matters staff, who knew that part of their role was to try to understand and address patients' needs and to recognize the relationships that were vital to them.

Rev. Marshall's experience visiting a severely ill patient revealed how these vital relationships influence a patient's experiences and decisions. When he entered the patient's room, he asked her how she was feeling and what she was thinking about. As he went to sit down on a chair with casters, it slid out from under him, leaving him sprawled out on the floor. Without making any acknowledgement of his fall or his position on the ground, she started talking about her son's divorce and her grandchild. The patient was crying because her daughter-in-law told her that she would never see the child again. Rev. Marshall got up off the floor and back onto his seat as she continued talking. He explained how a patient's focus is often directed not towards their illness, but toward their relationships:

> Her tears flowed. My well-being was not that important at the moment [*laughter*]. But it also was not about her serious health issue. She did not talk about that at all. What was most important to her was this relationship that she had with little Timmy. That is all that mattered to her. It was what she was focused on.
>
> A lot of end-of-life conversations go the same way. Family is who they are focused on. People will get up, and they live on for their grandchildren and their great-grandchildren, or whoever. And when we recognize that importance, and when we give a person reverence and elevate that relationship, that is when we connect with people.

We often hear an aging parent tell their family that they do not want their own health issues to be a burden for them. On many occasions a child or loved one discovers that the patient kept their unwelcome medical news secret so as not to upset them. This desire to protect loved ones is often interpreted by incredulous healthcare providers as proof the patient is making poor or irrational choices. Yet in the mind of the patient, it is the most rational choice.

One such case involved Jonah, an elderly African American man who had an inoperable tumor that was increasingly blocking his respiratory tract. Alert and oriented x 3 (to person, place, and time), the patient was approached about transitioning to hospice. But Jonah was adamant that he wanted everything possible to be done, including full resuscitation if needed. Staff made many visits to his bedside, hoping he would consent to the morphine he would need to help with the inevitable respiratory struggle. Martha was assigned to this case:

I had a good rapport with the patient's son, who totally understood that the staff's goal was to help his father ease into death, and that we needed his father's OK to move to comfort measures. His son opened an important door of understanding for me in one of our talks together. He explained that his father had been a fighter his whole life. That was his approach to life and the way he faced the world each day. His father had taken on the responsibility of raising two young grandchildren, and he took that responsibility seriously. He said, "How could my father give up? How could he, after his whole life of fighting for what he believed was the right thing to do, allow himself to say, 'I quit'? It would go against everything he had fought and stood for."

Jonah's decision may seem counterintuitive to healthcare providers, but the lesson that it teaches needs to be recognized and understood: the important relationships in a patient's life are integral to their deeply held beliefs and the decisions that they make.

Representing the patient's voice

Gail and Family Matters staff experienced every possible combination of family members. There were patients with large families that included siblings, spouses, adult children, and adult grandchildren. There were patients who had only one remaining family member, maybe the spouse or an adult child. There were patients whose only remaining relatives were nieces and nephews that had not been in the picture for years, or maybe ever. There were elderly patients who had lived independently with just friends or neighbors visiting and helping them.

Family Matters was frequently consulted to help the medical team identify the appropriate family member who would be the medical decision-maker if the patient were no longer capable. When a patient is competent, identifying a spokesperson is as simple as asking the patient who they would like their spokesperson to be, which is commonly done on admission. But if patients are confused, have dementia, or are medically compromised, they cannot reliably name who they would want to make decisions on their behalf if necessary.

This task was particularly important when there was a large group of family members, a family that was not in consensus with each other about medical decisions, or when there was no family at all.

Gail remembers her largest family meeting. It was for the matriarch of a Latino family. The meeting took place in a conference room with Gail and the attending physician. Tables and chairs were set up in a large square, and 22 people were in attendance. The striking aspect of this family, one that made an impression on Gail, was that every member at the family meeting knew of the patient's wishes and under what conditions she would want her treatment to stop. The patient had openly talked about her end-of-life wishes, and the whole family was there to make sure everyone respected her wishes.

If every family was as in sync with the patient's wishes and with each other as this family, having a spokesperson may not be as important. However, in many cases the situation is more complex, and identifying a spokesperson is crucial to ensure the patient's wishes or best interests will be represented in the medical decisions that must be made.

Family challenges and conflicts of interest

When a patient is in critical condition, family members can emerge from the woodwork. It is the ethical duty of the hospital staff to ensure decisions are in line with the patient's wishes and are based on the most recent discussions.

In one Family Matters case, several adult children were not aware—until the emergency medical admission of their father—that they had half-siblings. The patient had several different IDs in his wallet when he was found unconscious. With the patient remaining unresponsive, it was important to work toward a consensus among his offspring regarding necessary medical decisions, and to support these young adults, who were dealing with more than they had ever bargained for.

Eileen Dunleavy, BSN, HCEC, RN, is a seasoned critical care nurse and clinical ethics consultant. She joined Oakwood's clinical ethics committee in 2003 and eventually became staff for the Clinical Ethics Consultation Service. The red-haired mother of five worked in critical care for many years and is a fierce advocate of a patient's right to self-determination.

"The key role of the family is to respect the wishes of their loved one," she said. "That is the key role."

However, conflicts can arise when a patient has not expressed their wishes regarding their treatment or who should make decisions for them. These conflicts can cause delays in care, extensions of non-beneficial treatments, breakdowns of communication on all levels, and fragmentation of the family unit.

In their ethnographic study on intensive care units, Quinn et al. (2012) describe how family members involved in medical decision-making often position themselves in informal roles, especially when the patient has a life-threatening illness. The authors argue:

> Jockeying for position in the family system can be viewed as a consequence of the removal, by life-threatening illness, of a member of the system and a scramble for a new status in that altered system. Thus, for example, with the removal of an ill parent, adult children might move to claim status and authority in the system previously held by that parent (p. 49).

The informal roles that Quinn et al. identified were:

- primary caregiver
- primary decision-maker
- family spokesperson
- patient's wishes expert
- healthcare expert
- out-of-towner
- protector
- vulnerable member of the family

The researchers concluded that healthcare providers greatly benefit from understanding these roles and developing strategies to work with the family members who have adopted them (Quinn et al., 2012).

A family member can take on one or more of these roles. For example, the spouse of a critically ill patient may not be the patient's *primary caregiver* and may not have had treatment conversations with him. Think of an elderly father cared for by his adult daughter. She is the one who showers him, prepares his meals, feeds him, gets him up in the morning, and puts him to bed at night. The patient's wife may be too ill to help her husband. The daughter believes she has the best understanding of his declining health, and that she should become the *primary decision-maker* if her father were unable to make decisions.

But her brother, the *out-of-towner*, may have a different opinion of what should be done based on the wishes his father had expressed to him in the past. He may also have a mindset that his role is to swoop in and "take charge" after he arrives to make up for his absence. Imagine that this son works in the healthcare industry and was his father's *healthcare expert.*

Both the daughter and the son consider themselves the *patient's wishes expert*.

Add to this mix another daughter who is a recovering alcoholic and has been in and out of the father's life. Family history casts her as a *vulnerable member of the family*. Her siblings do not want to tell her that their father is failing or include her in the decision-making. She is considered the wild card. But she also has a teenage daughter who is remarkably close to her grandfather and who would be devastated if she were not made aware of the critical nature of his illness.

Frequently, family members caution the medical team about a relative who had fallen out of grace for some reason and is deemed untrustworthy.

Rev. Marshall recalled a family member telling him, "When she gets here, she is the bad one." And before I know it, I am waiting for the bad one [*laughter*]. The woman is not bad. I just got pulled onto that side."

The various family roles are not necessarily permanent. They will often shift and change with the circumstances. In nature, the goose that is the leader of a formation will drop back as it tires and let another goose take its place. Sometimes the leader of the family unit is the patient herself who has suddenly become critically ill, which forces others to step into unfamiliar roles. Many variations of the family dynamic can occur as the group seeks to stabilize.

It is important for healthcare providers to recognize how family dynamics can delay or influence decision-making. Eileen Dunleavy learned through her years of experience that sometimes a family member who comes across as a protector of a vulnerable patient is motivated by their own self-interest:

> There is a common denominator that I see. I cannot relate to it, but I understand it. It is often with middle-aged men who still live with their moms. Men that do not necessarily have a career or occupation and have lived in that house their entire life and have never had to work and get a job. When you have this family dynamic, it is often the same story. The son does not know what to do without his mother. He realizes that when the mother's death occurs, the house will be sold and divided between the other independent siblings. His home will be gone. His income will be gone. It influences his decisions for life-prolonging treatment for his mother and often does not align with the patient's wishes. He might know that it influences his decisions, but it is such a tug.

In cases like these, a decision to end life-sustaining care will have life-changing consequences for family members. These scenarios illustrate the need for staff to have a contextual understanding of the family dynamics, especially regarding who is the spokesperson.

Sometimes the adult dependent child is the only family member and decision-maker. In such cases it is particularly important to account for the parent-child relationship and to be aware of any wishes the patient may have expressed. Family Matters staff learned that it was often difficult for a family member to suspend their own preferences or values and make decisions based on the patient's best interests or desires.

Gail described an "aha" moment when she gained a new understanding of the forces that can influence decision-makers:

> It is a case about a patient I will call "Charlie." He must have been in his 70s and a very brittle diabetic, insulin dependent with gangrene of the feet. They had to start amputating his leg, and it was a tough story. They whittled away at his body, literally up to his knees and eventually up to the groin, so he was this half person. "Lisa May"

was his wife, and she would come every day by taking two buses from Detroit to get there.

Family Matters got called in early on in this case. Charlie already had a below-the-ankle amputation when I first got involved. The doctors still had treatments to offer, but they kept whittling away, and eventually he got septic. His wife came in every single day. She would just sit there and hold his hand. The doctors would sit down with her, and they would communicate about Charlie's medical diagnosis/prognosis. Other healthcare providers would come in as well and try to reinforce the information. It just got to be so futile, and Charlie was so septic the next step was going to be full intubation and ICU. By this time, he had just half a body.

It was then that the case became one for the ethics team. I remember going up to the room every day, sometimes twice a day and spending time with his wife. She would stay all day. I would try to open the conversation by asking her what the doctors told her about what was going on and see if they were keeping her informed. I asked if there was anything she did not understand. She would say, "Oh, I understand everything." It got really bad, and the gangrene was spreading.

We were all frustrated. The doctors and I needed her consent to stop aggressive treatment. We tried to help her to understand that there was no hope for Charlie, and it was not that we were just giving up and letting him go or letting him die.

One day I was losing my patience. I went up there, and she was standing holding his hand, and I was on the other side of the bed and looking at him. I almost had a tear in my eye, and I asked her, "Why are you doing this? He is dying. Would he have wanted to live this way?"

She just started crying and sobbing. Five minutes later she calmed down. She said, "Gail, I do not know what to do." She started crying again, and I asked her how we could help her. She said, "I live on his Social Security. What am I going to do?"

To me it was a "bingo" moment. We immediately got the social workers involved. They should have been involved before, but she never shared that detail because she was ashamed.

It was a big reason for her to keep Charlie alive. Huge. Once we got a social worker in to help her and she knew she was going to be OK, we let him go and kept him comfortable. She was there, and I was there. It was not a great death, but it was a better death than what would have occurred had we started to put tubes into every orifice of his body. I think talking about that scenario finally got through to her, and then she revealed that she was scared because she thought everybody was going to forget about her. There were no other family members. He was all she had.

You can almost empathize with that reasoning. What a lonely life.

Often the chronic illness of a patient will extend over many years and family members will take turns in the roles they play. But exhaustion, stress, and personal burdens take a toll over time, and when decisions about limiting treatment in the final stages of an illness arise, family differences often become more pronounced.

If family consensus unravels, it can have a profound effect not just on the family itself but also on the patient's care. In one Family Matters case, a patient had told one of his adult children that he would not want aggressive care when recovery was no longer possible. When the patient was no longer competent to decide, there was such a conflict among the four adult siblings and their spouses that a consensus decision could not be reached, even with multiple family meetings.

The family eventually went to court to seek guardianship. The intent was that one of them would be granted the right to be the legal spokesperson to make medical decisions for their father. But the animosity among the siblings, and the conflicting accounts they presented, prompted the judge to bypass all of them and appoint a public guardian. The guardian had no prior relationship with the patient but was still deemed better able to make decisions in the best interest of the patient. In the siblings' struggle for each to become the one with the power to make decisions for their father, they all lost.

Honoring the significance of relationships in self-determination

In their article "Translating psychosocial insight into ethical discussions supportive of families in end-of-life decision-making," Foster and McLellan (2002) discuss how end-of-life decision-making is an inclusive family process that has not only a clinical but ethical dimension that centers "on the moral realm of give and take between family members revealing fundamental questions about guilt, responsibility, and commitment to end-of-life care and decisions" (pp. 41-42).

One of the best ways to ensure that a patient's choices are honored is by making it a priority to discuss personal preferences while the patient can still express them. The benefits of completing an advance directive cannot be overstated, and making the effort to create one should be considered both the patient and the family's responsibility.

It is important for healthcare providers to recognize that sometimes the patient may choose to meet the needs of loved ones ahead of self-interest. One Family Matters case involved a woman who, on her deathbed, asked to be kept alive in the hope that it would bring her dysfunctional family together. There were numerous cases in which a terminally ill patient chose to continue burdensome treatment because a family member did not want them to give up. And so, respecting autonomy also entails understanding the importance of relationships, and to what lengths a person may go to put others before their own comfort.

After all, family relationships do not end at the hospital room door, and the importance and influence of family ties do not diminish in the face of a serious diagnosis. As Dr. Weber notes, "Alone and independent is not our model of a good citizen, a good family member, or a good person. It is rather that we are part of a larger unit."

Ideally, the family unit is held together by individuals who support each other, honor each other, and can assist each other. Father Richard Leliaert, PhD, who served for many years as Oakwood's healthcare chaplain and a manager of Spiritual Support Services, shared what he described as a "truly wonderful" experience in the story of his father's illness and the role family played in the decisions made at the end of his life:

> Way before I even came to Oakwood, even got into healthcare, my dad died. My dad died of kidney disease. He was a football player in his young days, and they had no protective equipment. He was a running back. An incredibly good one. I am not biased but my sister and I were awed at how good he was.
>
> So over the years he developed a more serious kidney problem. Then came the point in the late 1970s that Dad was just past retirement in his mid-to-late 60s, and he began to develop very severe kidney problems which required dialysis. And at that time, considering autonomy,

Dad did not want to undergo dialysis. But my mother, who he called Lou, asked him, "Would you just undergo dialysis even though you don't want to?" And I remember, God love him, [him] saying "Lou, only for you."

So, Dad let go of his autonomy for the sake of my mother. And because of that we had a remarkable nurse who picked up Dad three times a week to take him to dialysis. My mother went with them. That was a kind of happy time in Dad's life, even though he did not really appreciate dialysis. So, it came to be maybe about three years into dialysis, Dad began to see a lot of people dying, and he himself was beginning to feel that he was coming to the end of his rope, if you will. He just simply said to my mother, "Lou, no more." And God love my mother, [she] said, "I love you and will honor that." The family's experience was truly wonderful.

The "me" and the "we"

Father Leliaert had many roles during his career—educator, priest, hospital chaplain, ethics committee member, and administrator. Though he may not have encountered all the challenges and nuances of incorporating family in the care of the patient, he had a profound understanding of the family's influence and often its indivisibility.

Father Leliaert's experiences led him to advocate for a harmonious balance of patient and family needs:

[In the early part of my career,] we did value autonomy. It was a very, very big thing. And I think we bent over backwards, especially legally, to make sure that the patients' rights were not withheld or tampered with or bullied. But I thought the problem with that was…that we tended to put legality and ethics almost on similar rails, and that we were beginning to think that taking care of the legal side of it and taking care of the ethical side were the same thing. So, that presented a problem for me because legality should not be identified with ethics. I think that ethics should even be broader than legality.

What I learned the most was an old thing that we used in teaching the people in managed care. I developed this little model of the ME and the WE. If you look at a capital M, E, ME [it signifies] autonomy: my "ME-ness" and my rights. But if you turn the capital M upside down, you get a W, for the "WE-ness."

I think the role of an ethics committee in those days was how to help show the families, especially the person that was dying, or the person who is very ill, how their ME-ness could flow in the life of the WE-ness and vice versa. If that circle, I call it "circle of life," is really flowing then whatever decisions we made did more than protect us from lawsuits. It brought a state of being in which ethical principles and family relationships could have the best possible end result.

Yes. The ME-ness and the WE-ness. If you put too strong a line between them, you get individualism, which is not healthy. But I think God designed both our individuality, our unique ME-ness, made in His image, which nobody, nobody can take from us—and our WE-ness, our relationship in communion with others, including the family community, the hospital community, and the community at large.

I believe our ethics committee by and large was very instrumental in helping families achieve that ideal in the best way possible.

Join our Circle

- In Martha's experience, the most important thing to remember when working with patients and their families is showing them that you care and that you are listening. **What are some ways that you have demonstrated your concern and support to the families that you have worked with?**

- Mary Catherine helped her hospice patient talk to her husband about her impending death. **Has there ever been a time that you played a role in helping a patient communicate with family members about a sensitive or difficult topic? How did you feel when you took on this role?**

- The study by Quinn et al. identifies informal roles that family members can take on when they are involved in medical decision-making. Being aware of these roles can help healthcare providers better understand family dynamics. **What do you do to gain a better understanding of how family members relate to the patient and to each other? Can you recognize the roles your own family might play if one of you were to fall critically ill?**

- Conflict can arise when families become involved in medical decision-making, especially when it involves serious or life-threatening illnesses. **What experiences have you had with addressing and mitigating family conflict within the hospital setting?**

Chapter 4

Closing the Circle when Cultures Collide

We see things not as they are, but as we are.

—H.M. Tomlinson

Just as patients' families are often integral to their medical decision-making, a patient's cultural background can also have a significant impact on how they approach their medical care.

During much of her career, Gail worked at Oakwood Hospital in Dearborn, Michigan. Dearborn is a city of 103,000 that shares a border with Detroit. Its unique cultural evolution offered valuable lessons for the healthcare providers at Oakwood, requiring them to reflect on their own cultural attitudes and beliefs as they administered care to others.

While the examples we offer in this chapter primarily reflect Dearborn's large Muslim population, our country's changing cultural landscape makes it likely that you too will experience the challenges and rewards of working with a diverse patient population during your healthcare career. In this chapter, we discuss how our colleagues approached culture as an important dimension of their patients' medical decision-making and end-of-life experiences.

It is essential for healthcare providers to be aware of the diverse cultures that exist within a hospital's patient population because cultural beliefs can affect how patients view medical information and treatment options. It's equally important for providers to recognize how their own cultural background informs their perspective and understand how it interacts with patients' cultural beliefs. Being conscious of these cultural influences allows providers to break through impasses to communication and trust, creating a starting point for mutual understanding and respect.

Dr. Haydon recalls how his journey toward greater cultural awareness began:

> From the time I stepped into kindergarten until I finished medical school, I was this proud child who did well in school and was going to be a doctor. It was your typical nuclear middle-class family. I enjoyed and got a lot of praise for my academics, and I also did well in sports, so I kind of had an ego. My mother would always try to bring me back to planet Earth and would say, "Everybody has something important for you to learn from, everybody, so listen to everybody."

> I was somewhat shielded from the real world in many ways…I never really was out into the world and then I came to Dearborn. In thinking about it, when I was confronted by such diversity it stopped me in my tracks because of my traditional upbringing.

Dr. Haydon admits his limited worldview took a decisive pivot once he began practicing at Oakwood, which he described as "being all over the map" and much different from his own cultural upbringing:

> And I think I struggled with that when I first started. My take-home lesson was…you really had to be empathetic. You really had to understand another position. So, I think it was that spiritual, cultural, and religious diversity at Oakwood that forced me to kind of understand that. And [how important it is that] once you start seeing things from another perspective, just like ethics in general, that there is more than one right way to view things. And if, unfortunately, you come into some kind of conflict… rather than be arrogant about it and just say, "My way

is the right way" and "To hell with everybody; I'm not listening," it causes you to stop. As I remember it, there were some great people who were trying to do the right thing here. I think that is when we all started to get together and say, we need a more organized format to try to tie in these cultural differences.

Gail, the CECS staff, and the ethics committee members learned how cultural diversity could positively or negatively affect the patient-provider relationship, especially with end-of-life care decisions. The ethics committee sponsored educational presentations for the hospital staff about cultural diversity and reviewed new policies that were being formulated to accommodate the changing hospital population.

These efforts were necessary because over the last 50 years, Dearborn, Michigan, the home of Oakwood Hospital and Medical Center, saw major shifts in its population. In the 1970s, Dearborn, which shares a border with Detroit, was known for its history and legacy of racism and racial exclusion. Oakwood's patients and the residents of Dearborn were then primarily White, but things began to change. Martha remembers:

> I worked on the medical floor as a new graduate nurse in 1975. At that time, each patient on the units had a card that listed all their essential information like their diagnosis, diet, level of activity, planned treatments and overall nursing care plan. It also included the patient's nationality and religion. At that time, a significant number of the patients on my floor were listed as Polish and Catholic. In 2005, when I returned to work in the hospital, not only the patient population but also a substantial percentage of the staff were from the Middle East.

The Muslim population grew as Middle Eastern immigrants continued to arrive in Dearborn. By the 1990s, Dearborn became one of the largest Arab communities outside the Middle East and is presently the largest concentration of Arab American people in the United States. In addition to the growing Muslim community, many Arab immigrants are Lebanese Chaldeans, a culture that speaks Aramaic and practices Eastern Rite Catholicism.

Along with Dearborn's changing population, its status as a teaching hospital brought in many international residents, creating a culturally diverse staff that helped facilitate a more multiethnic environment for patients. Oakwood's healthcare force included providers from Central America, South America, India, the Middle East, Eastern Europe, the Philippines, and Asia.

Spiritual diversity at Oakwood

I think the institutions that are doing well recognize the need for spiritual support. Those that rank as top hospitals usually have a good spiritual support program and a strong clinical pastoral education program because they realize that people are more than just the bodies that we are in. If we are going to serve people, we must connect to them emotionally and spiritually.

—Reverend Doctor Tony Marshall

In addition to its efforts to support cultural diversity, Oakwood's administration and medical staff also fostered spiritual diversity. By educating staff, developing resources and tools, and building protocols into hospital policy, they helped create an environment that recognized and attended to the spiritual needs of all faith backgrounds. For example, instructional sheets were made available for staff in all the units outlining the protocol for critically ill Muslim patients, such as having their beds positioned to face towards Mecca, the direction that devout Muslims face to pray five times daily. For a Muslim, facing Mecca from wherever you are located signifies worldwide unity and reverence to the Kaaba, a monument said to be the "House of Allah."

Oakwood also adopted a policy for patients who are Jehovah's Witnesses. Because Jehovah's Witnesses view blood transfusions as a sin that is against God's will, the policy required a Family Matters staff member to consult with the patient upon admission. In the event that a transfusion became medically necessary, staff needed to obtain clarification from each patient about their specific limits or allowances for receiving blood or blood products. Most Jehovah's Witnesses had a legal document regarding blood transfusion restrictions which became part of their medical record. Their chart was flagged to alert the medical team.

Other measures were taken to promote religious understanding. The ethics committee hosted imams, Jehovah's Witnesses elders, rabbis, and other faith leaders inviting them to speak at their quarterly educational sessions. Shama Mehta was the first Buddhist chaplain to become part of the diverse staff and volunteers that made up Oakwood's Spiritual Support Department. Oakwood also renovated its chapel to allow both a Muslim prayer space and a meditation area that included expressions of Christian faith, such as a crucifix and bible.

Putting these protocols and resources in place did not happen without growing pains, and there were many challenges along the way. But as different spiritual disciplines learned and worked together, staff became more aware of the many ways people find meaning in their lives and in the world. By recognizing how essential spiritual identity can be to a person and finding ways to honor that, Family Matters staff were able to better assist Oakwood patients in closing the circle.

Father Richard Leliaert, PhD, and Reverend Doctor Tony Marshall, DMin, are two Oakwood chaplains who experienced the hospital's changing culture. When Father Richard started at the hospital, Oakwood was primarily composed of White Christian patients. Rev. Marshall, who arrived later, was Oakwood's first African American chaplain when African Americans were a minority of the staff and patient population.

As part of Oakwood's Spiritual Support Department, they were asked for assistance during many healthcare crises, but Rev. Marshall estimated end-of-life cases made up the majority of their interventions.

Father Richard Leliaert, PhD

Father Richard is currently a retired priest in the Archdiocese of Detroit. He has served as a priest for 53 years in three main capacities: as a college professor of religious studies, as a healthcare chaplain and manager of spiritual support at Oakwood, and as a parish pastor in a nearby suburb. While he was at Oakwood, he was also co-chair of the Oakwood Healthcare System's Corporate and Clinical Ethics Committees, serving as a member of its Transcultural Strategic Committee with a special focus on Muslim and Hispanic populations. He served the hospital from 1993 to 2005.

His role as a hospital chaplain followed 20 years as an educator. His love of learning and teaching stayed with him, and he frequently peppers his speech with lessons on the roots of words: "I like to use the word 'confluence.' It's from Latin, from things flowing together with other things. The word 'clinical,' as you know, comes from a Greek word, *klina*, which means 'bed.'"

Father Richard was at Oakwood "at a marvelous period of its growth." He credits the hospital's long-standing CEO, Gerald Fitzgerald, for supporting the development of transcultural efforts as Oakwood's population changed, stating, "God love him, when Jerry was there, I always felt that pastoral care would be safe and in a good way." He reflected on Oakwood's successful outreach to its Muslim community:

> Oakwood was outstanding. I do not think there was any other hospital in the whole country that did what we did to care for our Muslim population.
>
> Cultural things make a difference. We lump together all ethnic groups, and it is a mistake. But there is something that I call an intensity of values that is more prominent in one group than another. For example, in Islam, you really must sense what is a value to them. It's not just an obligatory collecting and acknowledgment but trying to be with them. Put your feet in their shoes. This is so important, whether you agree with them or not.

Even though there was a set protocol for what actions to take when a Muslim patient was dying, Father Richard knew that spiritual care was more than checking an item off a to-do list. Positioning a Muslim patient's bed to face east toward Mecca might have been a cultural protocol for staff to follow, but for the patient and family it was a spiritual dictate required by the Almighty.

Father Richard believes that if the hospital staff lacks understanding of the reasons for a patient's behavior, the opportunity to connect with them at a deeper level is lost:

> There was a time when our nursing staff was a little bit too, not rigid, but they would say, "Oh, we know all of that; we have already done that, been there, done that. We positioned the patient facing east."
>
> We do not do harm, let's face it, but we fail to reach the peak that we could if we were a little more attentive. Whether it is at the end of life or not, the totality of spiritual care and education is super important. But not just as another piece of information we tuck away. How do the practitioners of their faith live it out? It is important to understand

because that is what drives them. Muslim and Islam are not just concepts. It [is a way of life]. That is why in Islam, when you prostrate yourself, your whole body touches the ground.

The diversity among Oakwood's spiritual support staff was also present within religions. In Father Richard's work with Chaplain Schweib Gerguri, he observed that even within the same religion, there may be cultural barriers to overcome:

> The diversity within the Arab population was a learning experience as well. The chaplain, Sunni imam Schweib Shuaib Gerguri, was from Albania. He wore a suit instead of the traditional religious dress of the Shi'ite imams from the Middle East. So, when Schweib Shuaib responded to a request to visit a Muslim patient, they would complain, saying they were expecting a "real" imam. It took a while for me and Schweib Shuaib to work this out, but his patience and demeanor eventually made a great difference, especially in end-of-life or ethical consult situations.

Father Richard also recalled working with Eide Alawan, a member of Oakwood's ethics committee who served as a liaison between the Muslim population and the Dearborn community. Eide sat on other hospital ethics boards in Detroit. He was an important figure in a local mosque and was recognized as a pivotal part of helping others better understand the Muslim community. He was loved and admired by everyone who met him, and he interacted with all faith-based groups.

Father Richard's collaboration with spiritual leaders like these at Oakwood illustrates his belief that it is through authentic connections and relationships that we "reach the peak" of intercultural understanding. Cultural and spiritual diversity in the healthcare setting is not just a roster of the different cultures represented in a hospital and a list of their attributes and beliefs.

It takes more than collecting facts about cultural similarities or dissimilarities to provide effective spiritual support for diverse populations. It means acknowledging there is a "why" behind these differences. It is what Father Richard refers to when he provides us with the etymology of the word "understand": its root meaning is to "stand in the midst of" or "stand close to."

Father Richard's dedication to achieving a deep understanding of others helped him provide invaluable spiritual support for Oakwood's diverse community. Like Gail, he had an instinctive sense of whom to hire to help him with this role, and Rev. Marshall fit the bill.

Reverend Doctor Tony Marshall, DMin

Rev. Marshall says that he "stumbled" into healthcare pastoral work. He trained to be in a full-time ministry, but an internship in clinical pastoral education led to a 25-year career in healthcare chaplaincy. He is currently Program Manager of the Michigan Medical Clinical Pastoral Education Program at Mott Children's Hospital.

According to Rev. Marshall, the biggest challenge in transitioning from being a pastor to being a chaplain in healthcare was working with a more diverse group of people. And while he acknowledges that the work is intriguing and exciting, he notes that it is also incredibly challenging:

> Every church has a doctrine, a dogma by which they stand and follow and are willing to die for. But that does not work in a chaplaincy. I have to be willing to open myself up to hear from others' perspectives. To feel what other people are feeling. To understand them and to engage them right where they are. To do that challenges my own beliefs and my own core values. So, I had to mature and be mature enough to open myself up to that. Part of that is

the training process, but a lot of it comes from experience and meeting wonderful people who are Muslim, Catholic, Hindu, Buddhist, or "Nons" as we say sometimes, and seeing the beauty and spirituality in their lives as well.

I want to come in with an open mind to meet them where they are and to get some information. "What are you experiencing?" "Where do you see, if you see God, involved in the process?" When we talk about spirituality, it is a question about what is most important and what is most dear…I have seen a lot of people who really aren't afraid of dying. They just do not want to leave their family members. That is what becomes most important to them. Well then, I will meet them at that place. So, I think it is very important that we meet people where they are and find out where they are, what is important to them, and what means the most to them.

Even though every chaplain trains to serve whomever needs spiritual support, there were times Rev. Marshall was specifically requested to see a patient or family because they were African American. Rev. Marshall believes that connecting with others on the basis of heritage is one of many ways to connect:

If you say race should not make a difference, well, yes and no. I believe in the beauty of all ethnicities and genders and all that we are. And in saying that, I do not want to become a nothing. I am an African American man and I hold distinction in my being and in being framed in that person. So, if I become nothing, just an entity, then I would lose that beauty. I would never want to lose my African American heritage, nor would I ask anyone else to lose his or her heritage. I believe that we can try to use these things. Let us not build them as barriers but let us use them as roads.

In Rev. Marshall's journey from a pastor to chaplain to head of a chaplaincy program, he learned both how to embrace the reality of distinctions among us and how to reach across them:

> I have been in a room with families that I knew had racist feelings toward Black people, but when their mom was dying, they hugged me and cried on my shoulder. Maybe a seed was planted there, and maybe they would be different people tomorrow, but what took place in that moment is all that was important. I do not look at them and say, "You didn't speak to me in Kroger." That is not what I am here for. I threw my arms around them, and we prayed together, and I serviced the family as best as I could.
>
> One thing that I would add to our discussion is the universal aspect of death and dying and grief in this work. We see patients that come from all the economic and social statuses of life, especially in a place like this. But it is the same denominator. When the end of life comes up, we are all the same.
>
> I have seen all kinds. I have worked with families that did not speak English at all, but their grief is the same thing. It is one of those elements of life that we all deal with. It brings back, I think, that true humanity, that true brotherhood and sisterhood of all, Dr. King's Beloved Community. We are all the same when it comes, so it does not matter whether you are from the White House or living on the street. Grief and death and dying, end-of-life is universal. That is one of the reasons I think we can come together and help one another, and that is the beauty of it. I wish we could take that type of thinking beyond those walls. We seem to have trouble with that.

Cultural diversity in the delivery of healthcare

In the early stages of Oakwood's cultural changes, its administration created the Transcultural Strategic Task Force, a trailblazing effort headed by Najah Bazzy, RN, and Rose Khalifa, RN, who pioneered educational initiatives to build a culturally competent workforce. The task force provided a model that other departments used to develop their own cultural competency training.

Moe Rustom's cultural background and clinical experience made him well-equipped to deliver culturally competent healthcare. When he joined Family Matters Support Service, he quickly became the point person for culturally sensitive cases.

Mohamad (Moe) Rustom, MSA, RN, FACHE

Mohamad, or Moe, as he was both respectfully and amicably called, is an Arab American who played a significant role in helping staff understand the traditions of Arab culture. His own personal experience with cultural diversity helped to pave the way:

> When I left Lebanon, I was very close-minded. I was an idiot. I thought the world was very small until I went to Abu Dhabi, and there I met the Scottish, the Irish, the Welsh and a multitude of nationalities, including Americans. It was like whoa, whoa! You either embrace that difference, or you stand your ground and fight it all your life.

Trained as a registered nurse in Lebanon, Moe came to the United States and eventually to Dearborn, where he worked in Oakwood's emergency room. It was there that Gail and Chris met and sized up Moe, liked what they saw, and recruited him to be part of their team.

Moe soon became an asset to Family Matters and the SCEC. Eventually, Gail encouraged Moe to branch out on his own. Having witnessed the importance of effective communication in serving Oakwood's diverse patient populations, he established the Clinical Language Service (CLS) Department and was appointed department head in 2005. Not only did this department serve the needs of non-English-speaking patients, but it also provided interpreters for people who were deaf, blind, and disabled.

The Clinical Language Service was a part of everyday operations at Oakwood, providing on-site interpreters trained in Spanish and Arabic, and two-receiver phone handsets that simultaneously connected both a patient and a staff member to certified interpreters in multitudes of other languages. These services allowed patients to receive information in the language they best understood so they were equipped to comprehend and discuss the many choices they were called upon to make around treatment options. Moe believed this service was essential for good healthcare. He always referred to Nelson Mandela's words: "If you talk to a man in a language he understands, that goes to his head. If you talk to him in his language, that goes to his heart."

Holding discussions with non-English-speaking patients and families can be a challenge for healthcare providers. When even one member of the team does not comprehend the communication, it can affect the delivery of healthcare. Chris personally experienced this challenge: "I think it is especially difficult because we have a lot of Arabic-speaking physicians and Arabic-speaking families. I am the one who needs the interpreter, so I know what everybody is saying."

In his role as Director of Clinical Language Services, Moe helped hospital staff recognize the culturally sensitive nature of communicating medical information to patients and families who were not proficient in English. He understood that it takes more than a direct translation of words to establish trust across different languages and cultures. Instead, an effective interpreter conveys the full meaning of the message. According to Moe, "The true measure of a good interpreter is how well they can transfer emotions, not just words." He often found that interpreters at Oakwood needed to explain cultural norms and taboos to non-Muslim healthcare providers:

> Take, for example, when a doctor comes in and asks a woman of Arab or Muslim descent if she had sex before marriage. That is very insulting. Regardless of whether the person had or did not have a relationship, a person of that culture would be reluctant to answer a question about an action that is considered a sin. This is where the cultural brokering comes in. The role of the interpreter is to stop a misunderstanding and explain the context of why the question is being asked, rather than having the patient assume that the provider was insulting that person's sanctity of spiritual being.

Each encounter an interpreter has requires sensitivity, cultural awareness, and a willingness to work together with the healthcare provider to communicate effectively with the patient. A good interpreter avoids cultural taboos, instead finding more culturally appropriate ways to get the information the healthcare provider needs to administer appropriate medical care. Moe explains:

> Say, for example, a physician wants to tell a patient, "You have cancer." In the American culture it is quite common to convey a message between a doctor and a patient in a direct way. It is part of the American culture that a person has the right to know, and they will be the ones who decide things in their life. The way a message is delivered to somebody who has cancer and is of Arabic heritage is not the same. Since it is a collective society, the family role is key, and decision-making by the immediate family is warranted and expected. There are many circumstances where families often shield patients from this information and assume decision-making on their behalf. The justification for this action is often explained as a desire by

the family to protect the patient's well-being from further aggravating news and potential emotional distress that is usually accompanied by a diagnosis of cancer.

Another problematic question is, "Do you take drugs?" [Think about] the elderly lady who prayed for all her life, wore the hijab, went to Mecca, and became a Haj. She lived in that atmosphere of fearing God and fearing everything that is sinful. Then you come in and ask her if she is taking drugs! Now, there is a way to ask that question, but not the way it is asked on a form or the way the physician will typically ask it.

Cultural nuances like these can cause challenges for healthcare providers because of their professional obligations to deliver truthful information and achieve informed consent for treatment. The last part of this chapter will touch on some of these ethical challenges.

Moe took the lead in educating nursing staff and all hospital personnel about cultural differences by developing online diversity courses and providing in-person support and education. He was especially instrumental on the critical care floors when a patient was in serious condition or dying.

One ongoing issue that needed a resolution involved Arab families' lack of "rule following" related to the number of visitors allowed on a unit. In Oakwood's critical care areas, visitors were limited to immediate family, often with restricted times. Oakwood was not prepared for the Arab tradition of having many visitors in the room with the patient. Moe recalls nurses on the critical care floors having difficulty dealing with patients from Arab and Muslim backgrounds because numerous family members and friends visited the patient and often remained all day:

In the beginning, some nurses were very defiant and unaccommodating. I had to do reoccurring education to work toward a more positive outcome. The nurses would see

15 or 20 people in the waiting room and view the situation as, "There is an opposing family who is a lot of trouble." I would explain that this was a cultural thing. People in the neighborhood want to come in and check on their neighbor and pay respect to the ill. In Western culture, it is different, but in other cultures, it is the entire neighborhood that comes to visit because it is seen as a duty.

Moe's work raised cultural sensitivity around the issue and produced solutions based on a better understanding of the situation. Helping staff understand why a behavior occurred rather than labeling it as good or bad reduced the conflict. The healthcare team identified key family members and gave them the task of coordinating visits and relaying the hospital rules to the visitors.

During her work with Family Matters, Martha saw firsthand how cultural beliefs can impact end-of-life care when she worked with a loving, dedicated husband of a critically ill patient and the patient's attending physician. The patient had lingered in intensive care for several months on full life support. She was minimally responsive and in multiple organ failure:

> I had been the Family Matters support person for the husband during the whole hospitalization, visiting the bedside daily and listening to his worries as he watched his wife's ongoing plateau in critical condition. One day, the husband said to me, "I trust that the doctor will tell me when there is no more hope, and it is time to stop. If he thinks she won't recover, I wouldn't want her to go through this any longer."

But there was an issue the husband was not aware of, in that this highly trained and well-respected physician was Muslim, and it would be going against his own beliefs to suggest treatment be withdrawn. In Islam, although scholars have deemed the removal of life support permissible in certain cases, there is a strong religious conviction that life is a gift from God and actions that would end life are forbidden. In this particular case I knew the patient's spouse was Christian, and I believed unaware of this tenet of the Muslim faith. Because I had a good rapport with the physician, I relayed to him what the husband had told me. I asked the physician to please consider how his own religious beliefs could influence the continuation of the patient's treatments, and that the husband needed to know his religious perspective.

After he reviewed the chart, I watched the physician walk into the patient's room and have a long talk with the husband in private. Shortly afterward, orders were written for comfort measures and withdrawal of life support. This case was extremely moving for everyone involved. It serves as an example of how different perspectives must be recognized and communicated.

After the patient died, I went to the funeral home to pay my respects. I felt someone tap my shoulder and turned to see it was the patient's physician. He had also come to honor the relationship he had with the husband and his patient. It was a moment I felt the power and compassion of closing the circle.

Understanding the beliefs and practices of different cultures does not always translate into being able to change your own mindset or to easily turn your back on a belief that is part of your own culture. Moe often found himself sitting on a fence between his cultural values and those he had acclimatized to while working in U.S. hospitals. This trait made him an asset as a mediator and educator because he could be sympathetic to the challenges that come with diversity in healthcare delivery.

Cultural conflicts and ethical challenges

The healthcare team consulted the CECS regarding conflicts that arose from differing cultural perspectives. Two recurring conflicts often took place. One was determining who should be the decision-maker. The other, and most profoundly challenging, was determining when—or if—life-sustaining treatment should be stopped. These ethical dilemmas were particularly frequent with the Muslim population, but the same challenges can occur within any culture, including within the Christian and Jewish traditions.

Who is the decision-maker?

One of the most prized ethical principles in Western medicine is autonomy. Dr. Reitemeier, who served as Corporate Director of Clinical Ethics at Beaumont Health near the end of Gail's tenure, defines autonomy in relationship to rationality:

> Autonomy is the ability to, in a reasonably consistent and durable way, evaluate the prospects for your own life, realistically, and to engage in a self-directed plan of living. You can have a lot of reasons, motives, and objectives, quite varying, and all of those would be quite consistent with saying that you are making autonomous decisions. It has to be rational. But beyond rational, there are not a lot of requirements for autonomy. And if you can give consistent reasons, we have to take that seriously.

His definition highlights why conflicts occur between different cultures in healthcare. If reasonable behaviors are defined as actions that comply with the traditions and practice of one's own culture, who determines what is rational in a multicultural patient population?

The challenge of recognizing the medical decision-maker has become more complicated as the definition of family has evolved over time. However, this ethical challenge can also include situations involving a *competent* patient who, based on cultural practices, is not seen by their community as the person in charge of their own medical decisions. In some Muslim and Hindu cultures, the male spouse or eldest son of a female patient is the decision-maker. In other cases, the whole family is involved.

Ann Caulfield-Cook, PhD, LMSW, was the social work supervisor in the Care Management Department at Oakwood until, nearing Gail's retirement, she was asked to join the CECS. Ann became the CECS supervisor and SCEC administrator. Her background of over 40 years in mental health and a private therapy practice added a new dimension to the essential work that Gail had championed. Ann remembers an ethics consult she worked on that involved clarifying the decision-maker for an unconscious patient from a Muslim culture:

> The patient had a wife and an eldest son. While we assumed the eldest son would be the decision-maker from their cultural background, we were surprised when the son said he could not make the decision alone. The family's cultural tradition was not having the eldest son decide alone but with the community elders. The son was adamant he had to present the decision about treatment options to the elders, and the treatment team had to wait for their response.

Gail participated in cases where a family did not want a competent patient to be their own decision-maker and sometimes did not want the patient to even be informed of what was wrong with them. In these situations, to comply with the hospital's ethical and legal standards, the patient had to be asked if they were freely giving up their own right to decide and to whom they were giving decision-making authority. As ethicist Dr. Weber asserted, a family member saying "don't tell her" is not enough. It had to be clear that this was the patient's choice. If it was clear they were deferring decision-making to someone else, then this directive could be honored. Gail educated staff that it was important to revisit and reaffirm that the patient's decision did not change over the course of their hospitalization.

Even if healthcare providers were aware of different cultural practices, these differences could still cause moral or professional challenges. For Dr. Derek Bair, a specialist for high-risk newborns and premature babies, it is never the patient who is the decision-maker; it is the parent. He remembers a case in which a baby was going to die despite their best efforts to save it. A Middle Eastern father was the self-appointed decision-maker and did not want the mother to be told the baby was dying, nor did he want her to be present. He directed Dr. Bair to keep fighting and to keep trying to save the baby. The father said that he would tell the mother what she needed to know. However, the baby's mother was American and had been raised in the United States. Based on his experience and knowing the importance of closure, Dr. Bair acted on his belief that the mother should be with her baby in its last moments and sent the nurse to get her. It was only when the mother came into the room that the baby died.

When cultural conflicts challenged the medical staff about what to disclose or about who was making the decisions, Family Matters worked to support the staff, patient, and family. Communication and education were key for everyone involved in the patient's care. The goal was to reach a resolution that respected a patient's choices but did not compromise the medical professional's obligation to practice ethically.

When differences prolong the dying process

Modern technology offers us devices that keep body systems functioning. These devices have remarkable power to save lives. But sometimes, they blur the line between saving a life and merely prolonging the dying process.

For most loved ones, stopping treatment when it no longer offers a chance of recovery can be an extremely difficult decision to make. But in certain cultures and religious practices, the family cannot request that life-sustaining support be withdrawn, even in the direst of circumstances. Martha's experience with the Muslim physician and Christian couple demonstrated a resolution of this type of cultural conflict, but at Oakwood, this prohibition was often seen within Muslim families. Moe Rustom explains:

> Decision-making in the Western culture is approached as, "I have my own decisions to make. I have my own privacy, and that is why we have laws. I decide what is going to happen to me." The Muslim culture's view is that "God will decide for me."

> Yet, as a Muslim, when you come to the West, you are often asked to make decisions that might defy everything that you learned in your life. Decisions that defy all the principles and all the doctrines that you have been taught and struggled with. And that struggle does not stop with the immediate patient or their families; it also extends into the community. There is an understanding of how things should go.

> [Asking a family for permission to withdraw support] creates a situation where beliefs that people have had all their lives get tested, and it is suddenly thrown in their lap to decide about life and death for their loved ones. First and foremost, if they were to make a decision toward termination, it would be committing a sin and would mean

going to hell. On the other hand, if you decide to extend life, you are also faced with the fact you are extending their suffering for a long time. But they end up choosing not to commit the sin and not going against God's wishes.

That is the backbone of all the disagreements about limiting or stopping treatments. They occur because of our expectations in Western medicine for a person from a culturally different mindset to decide to stop treatment. But what we are really asking them to do is to either commit a sin or, as I call it, carry a burden. I used this line in many of my diversity presentations: is it committing a sin or carrying a burden? They end up having to choose one of those two choices.

New immigrants in particular often hold fast to their own cultural roadmap to help them navigate their new world, especially in times of stress and challenge. This phenomenon can result in cultural conflicts around end-of-life care even within the same family. In Moe's experience, different generations within an immigrant family can result in different viewpoints on end-of-life decision-making:

I will tell you another story that I use in my presentation to explain the first and second generations. This was a Muslim family. They were immigrants who came from overseas. They came with their children, who were teenagers at that time. The children eventually got married and had kids born in this country. So, I witnessed a discussion between the immigrant's son and grandson. The intensivist went to the bedside and explained what was going on and the options. This was after the patient had been there for a while, and the treatments were not effective. The son was saying to the doctor, "Do everything you can." The grandson was saying, "Hold on, why do you want him to suffer?" This is an example of everything that the culture brings to the doors of American medicine.

Working with a diversity of cultural beliefs in a hospital setting can be challenging. The clinical ethics department made recommendations that acknowledged diverse cultural practices but also clarified professional responsibility.

It is important to note that the intergroup conflicts a healthcare staff can encounter do not just occur between Western and non-Western cultures. Attitudes embedded in racial prejudice that can occur within any society can result in friction or even hostility. In these cases, the same rationale for following ethical principles must apply. Dr. Weber notes:

> I do not know whether this has come up at Oakwood, but in many places, it has, and regards a patient not wanting a care provider providing care for them if they are of a particular ethnic or racial or religious background. Because we have this confusion about our responsibilities and our accommodating patient's wishes, we tend to cave in.

> The only right response to that, I think, is to say that we do not make work assignments based on patients' preferences. We provide qualified professionals who care for you. We are going to do that. It sounds harsh, but that is the only way you can deal with equality. The only way you can deal with equal opportunity is in the workplace. The only way you can deal with racism. The only way you can deal with any of that is to take a stand.

> But we do not because we are somehow handicapped by this idea that if we take a stand, people do not like it, and we're insensitive. No, we are very sensitive to our responsibilities. It does not have to be done harshly; it can be done very sympathetically. But backing down, out of somehow an understanding that this is respectful, is not respectful at all. It's saying that I don't really believe in my principles. I will do what you want.

Respect: The key to cultural competence

All the challenges that cultural diversity can present in a healthcare system are impossible to address here. However, the experiences that occurred during Gail's time at Oakwood demonstrated something essential to Family Matters and the other healthcare staff there: despite all their differences, cultural practices do not, as Rev. Marshall eloquently expressed, change the universality of dying. Neither do these differences change the importance of bringing as much dignity and integrity as possible to the dying process to assist patients in achieving a good death.

Moe Rustom, along with Father Richard, Rev. Marshall, Dr. Weber, Gail Daly, and other Family Matters and healthcare staff, worked together to make cultural competence an expectation at Oakwood. As an experienced healthcare professional, an Arab American, and the face of Oakwood's cultural diversity program, Moe offers a profoundly valuable perspective on the most effective way to frame cultural diversity for healthcare providers:

> I feel that academically, the country does a very good job at educating people in medicine and healthcare about cultural competency in books. But that is similar to teaching my daughter how to swim by showing her how it is done in a book. Then I go, and I push her into the pool and say, "Swim!" That is what we do with the healthcare providers. We end up just dropping them in and they end up finding out for themselves. They go through bad experiences and do not address the issues of how you need to interact.

> Many of the cultural competency training courses that I have seen are really focused on educating you about what that culture is. That is not what is going to make you an expert on a culture. The point of cultural competency is to make you well aware of the differences so you can respect them. That is the silver lining and the bottom line for

cultural competency, because if you don't have respect for that difference, there are going to be problems.

If you do not have it in you as a provider, a respect for something that is very different from you, you are going to fall into issues. Now, this does not mean the responsibilities are sideways and someone should just alternate between both sides. People do carry a responsibility to respect the system in place and that also should be conveyed. But most people are not very knowledgeable about this until they are told they are violating something. I do not think people do it on purpose.

Communication is key. I think that is what made us so successful in critical care. All of us were trained in carrying the message in the right environment through the right vehicle to the specific person receiving it. That made a lot of difference.

Join our Circle

- Both Dr. Haydon and Moe Rustom found that once they left home and the "bubble" of their own cultural upbringing, they had to expand their worldview to adjust to a much greater degree of cultural diversity. **Have you experienced something similar in your own life or work? How did you adjust? What resources or programs are currently in place to support staff in providing culturally competent care at your workplace?**

- Holding discussions with non-English-speaking patients and families can be a challenge for healthcare providers. This is not only because of the language barrier, but also because of the culturally sensitive nature of communicating medical information. **Can you recall a time when you struggled to communicate with a patient or family due to linguistic or cultural differences? What did you do to overcome the challenges you faced?**

- Dr. Weber notes that sometimes patients will not want a healthcare provider to care for them if they are of a particular ethnic, racial, or religious background. **Have you ever witnessed or experienced a patient refusing care from a healthcare provider due to the provider's race, culture, or religion? How was it addressed and resolved?**

- Even when a healthcare provider is aware of both their own and their patient's cultural beliefs and practices, the differences between them can still cause moral or professional challenges. **Under what circumstances does respect for a culture's different norms become a moral dilemma for a healthcare provider? What should take place if this occurs?**

- Father Richard believes that it is through authentic connections and relationships that we "reach the peak" of intercultural understanding. **Were you ever in a situation when you felt that you were able to form an authentic connection with someone from a different cultural background than your own? How did it happen?**

Chapter 5

Death: Attitudes, Fear, and Anticipatory Grief

I'm not afraid of death; I just don't want to be there
when it happens.

—Woody Allen

When the shift towards death begins, the patient experiences a dying process that has a nature and rhythm of its own. Dying is physically demanding. The symptoms of the dying process, especially after a long chronic illness, can include shortness of breath, difficulty swallowing, bed sores or skin tears, confusion, anxiety, and discomfort. Even when medications alleviate these symptoms, the outward signs signaling that death is near can be disturbing for loved ones to witness.

Just like welcoming a human life into the world, watching someone departing from it is a highly charged emotional experience. In this chapter, we will explore attitudes and emotions towards death and the dying process. We'll also discuss how fear and stress compromise a person's reasoning, and what Gail's team learned about anticipatory grief.

Our beliefs start forming in infancy. They are generated from many sources, most notably family attitudes, the culture we are born into, spiritual teachings, and our interpretation of individual experiences that occur over time. Our beliefs help determine whom we trust, what we value, and how to function within our social units. We may not always be aware of them, but the beliefs we form affect our thought processes. These include the beliefs we have formed about death.

To help someone through an end-of-life experience, healthcare providers must understand that patients' beliefs about death will inform their attitudes, interactions and medical decisions. Healthcare providers also need to be aware of their own beliefs about death and how these beliefs influence their own actions and reactions when dealing with others. When a patient is dying, the healthcare provider's point of view and priorities may differ from those of a patient or family. Martha notes:

> As part of Family Matters, I came to realize I should not make assumptions about what sort of medical decisions make sense to the family of a dying loved one. In end-of-life cases, often the mindset of staff was that the family or spouse were making irrational choices to continue non-beneficial care based on an assumption that they "just don't get it." But often it wasn't about "not getting" how sick a person was. It was about something else. Something that has not yet been addressed or identified.

Preserving life or prolonging death?

Modern Western culture plays a significant role in creating barriers that prevent talking openly about death. In the face of death, many people find it difficult to express honest emotion and communicate any end-of-life wishes to those we love.

Gail witnessed death every day working in critical care units and the emergency room. Although many patients survived, she observed more deaths than the average person ever would. These experiences helped Gail realize why it can be so difficult to talk with patients about death:

> What is important to one person might not be important

to another person.

There may be some people who would accept being in a wheelchair, as we all know people that are, [but for some people that would be unacceptable]. It is about the values that are important to that person. It is not about my values or anybody else's, but about that individual person who is making healthcare decisions about themself. If the person was still able to talk, I remember using the phrase, "What are you hoping for, in terms of your recovery? What are you truly hoping for?"

A lot of times, it was something that wasn't even possible. Being able to talk with someone about death was a process because it is hard to deal with your own mortality and you need help along the way. There is a lot of denial in place for most of us.

Part of that denial that we often experience can be attributed to the advancement of medicine. Prior to WWII, deaths in the U.S. that were due to natural causes took place at home. However, improvements in medical technology resulted in higher success rates at curing illness, and those with life-limiting illnesses and critical diseases often went into the hospital for continued treatment. The advent of high-tech medicine saved lives by offering some a cure that allowed them to recover. But for those unable to be cured, the same treatment prolonged the dying process.

As Chris Westphal previously described, at the beginning of her nursing career there were no long-term care facilities where people went to live on life support. She believes that providing options when there is no hope for recovery obscures the reality of what is happening. Chris explains, "We have blurred the line of where natural life ends. We've kind of discounted natural life. It is like a natural life's ending isn't valued. We just keep things going artificially many times."

For example, a nephrologist's recommendation of dialysis to restore a patient's kidney function does not necessarily grant the patient's wish of returning to a normal life—if dialysis must continue for the rest of the patient's life. Three trips a week to the dialysis unit for a compromised and chronically ill person will certainly affect the life they once knew and, subsequently, the lives of their family members.

Treatments that are not curative but prolong life do have value in many circumstances. Yet employing such measures when other bodily systems are failing (circulatory, respiratory, neurological) is a distraction that can prolong pain and feed denial.

Hiding behind the curtain: Death in isolation

When more people began to die in the hospital rather than at home, it altered the experience of death both for individuals and family members. Moving the end of life to a foreign environment hid the action of dying. This change hindered the family's ability to care for the dying person and their opportunity to recognize the signs of the dying process.

People who are at risk of death from acute injury or severe or complicated chronic illness are often admitted to a critical or intensive care unit. These units have a noticeably different feel from a general medical floor. On the general medical floor, there is a lot of activity in the hallways. Medical assistants, nurses, physician consultants, therapy staff, dietary personnel, cleaning staff, family members, and medical carts create a buzz of activity that mimics the social networks and familiar activities of life. Patients can choose when to keep the room door open or close it for privacy. It is still a regulated environment, but it is associated with the possibility of a return to health, or at least improvement and discharge.

When a family visits a critically ill hospitalized patient in a critical care unit, they enter an overwhelming environment of machines, tubing, and beeping alarm systems. The delivery of the most sophisticated treatment takes place in a very regimented setting. The private rooms isolate the patient in their own world. The hallways are clear so emergency teams can quickly respond to medical crises such as cardiac arrests. Sounds come from machines rather than staff and visitors chatting in the hallways. Staff members are reserved and quiet out of respect for the grave medical status of those that have been admitted. The nurses closely monitor their assigned patients.

A critical care patient's connection with others is limited by the nature of the unit itself. Even the bed's metal side rails enclose the patient in a "don't touch me" box. It's not uncommon for family visitors to take a seat at the periphery of the room, only tentatively approaching the bedside.

The majority of Gail's professional practice was in critical care, and most of the interactions that Family Matters support staff had with families occurred in this setting. Gail described the early days of critical care nursing and visitation rules:

> In the beginning, the amount of time that a family could visit would be only 5 to 10 minutes. We restricted who could visit and how long the visits would last. The rules were set forth by the administration and it was not questioned. Initially it was considered a positive thing. It worked for the nurses who did not want to be interrupted from their multiple tasks assigned on a rigid schedule. It worked for the rounding physicians who wanted to review diagnostics and access a patient without family interference.

> Eventually, our unit moved to a self-governance model, and we changed the visitation rules so they were less restrictive. The current model in most hospitals today

includes family as a part of the healthcare team and encourages their presence, but there were many years that this was not the case.

Even when a hospital has a family-centered approach, once someone is admitted, be they a mother, son, or spouse, they become "the patient." The hospital practices that go along with this new status can insulate the family from the severity of the patient's illness: crowded by machinery, supported by pillows, positioned comfortably, cleaned and covered, even a dying person can look good.

The healthcare team's use of medical jargon to describe the patient's status further obscures the reality of the dying process. In fact, the language of medicine is as inscrutable as the crisp white sheet that covers the declining body. When dying is physically hidden and medical terms camouflage difficult realities, a patient or family is sheltered from the information they need to process what is happening.

Although there have been great advancements with hospice and palliative care in returning the dying process to a family-centered environment, the act of dying remains largely hidden within hospital walls, lacking social recognition and acceptance as a natural and normal process. Palliative and hospice care providers acknowledge that when serious illness and the dying process occur in the hospital, it is difficult for families to recognize. Unfortunately, when a family finally does realize that the patient is dying, the opportunity to find closure with their mother, father, or loved one seems frantic and short.

Martha recounted a story of a family's attempt to find closure and connection in the foreign environment of a hospital room:

> Sara was dying. Her husband of 50 years and the 13-year-old grandson they were raising were both at her bedside. She had been unable to respond for the past couple of

days, and her death was close. Her husband and grandson stood, one at each side of the bed, like figures frozen in the moment. It was a crowded semi-private room, and they were trying to be polite visitors. But they wanted to say goodbye, and like two cats, they were waiting for the right moment to spring. Because of my experience with end-of-life support, I recognized their dilemma. I told them, "If you stay right by her, I will let the side rails down." I also drew the privacy curtain around the entire bed and stepped outside of it.

Although they were hidden from my sight, I heard them as they leaped into action. "I love you, Grandma" was repeated over and over again. The curtain moved as the bed shifted and I envisioned Sara's grandson holding her. Then came the click, click of a camera that must have been hidden in her husband's overcoat. His voice was soft and low, and I imagined him whispering in her ear and stroking her hair. They were reclaiming her as their own in the only way that seemed allowable. Standing outside of the curtain, I thought about how many times other families had felt they were not given permission to say goodbye in privacy, and in a way that was meaningful for them.

Addressing the "D-word"

Just as the act of dying is frequently hidden in our modern society, discussions about death and dying are often avoided. In some cultures, people hesitate to talk about death or even say the word "dying" because they believe that discussion of death invites the event itself to take place. In many cultures, it is often the case that families don't want their loved ones to know they are dying. They believe that this information should be kept a secret to protect the dying person from fear and a loss of hope. But this can also serve as a delaying tactic for the family members who are not ready to accept what is taking place or who don't know how to talk about it.

Healthcare providers can also be reluctant to talk about death. It is well documented that physicians who are trained in saving life are not trained in having end-of-life discussions. Many physicians admit that they have difficulty switching from conversations about saving life to conversations about comfort measures. This can happen because the relationship physicians have with their patients is based on trust and a promise (the ethical principle of fidelity) that they will do all they can to preserve the patient's life.

In his 40 years of experience in private practice, Dr. Hnatiuk experienced this dilemma when his patients needed end-of-life care:

> I saw my role as treating the patient in the hospital to try to get the patient home. Not to the funeral home. It is also very difficult for physicians most of the time to know that this is the end, this is all we can do. I have known this patient for years and years and now I'm going to have to let go of him or her.
>
> I think most physicians are uncomfortable discussing death, and they should be because it's not something you really enjoy doing. But they are also not trained in it. I do not remember taking any course on how to talk to a patient's family about death and dying and what decisions they may want to make.
>
> That is part of the discomfort: not knowing how to talk about it. There is no class for it. No right or wrong way of doing it, I suppose. Should there be? Probably. "How to talk to a patient" should be a class in medical school because there are physicians who graduate who do not know how to talk to a patient. If not in medical school, maybe as part of the internship or residency program. They should be required to go to these family meetings, discussions with the primary care physician or intensivist or whoever is making that discussion happen.

There is an art to medicine. Medicine is an art. Fifty percent art, probably, and fifty percent science. It is the communication part of the art that is missing and difficult to learn.

Jacqueline Mohs, MD, is a palliative care specialist. Her journey toward medicine began after spending two years in South Africa with the Peace Corps. On her return she pursued her medical degree and was drawn to geriatrics and then palliative care. Dr. Mohs frequently works with patients whose life-limiting illness is no longer curable. Her patients' serious or terminal medical status and the nature of her work requires her to have end-of-life conversations more frequently. General practitioners or internists may be less familiar—and less comfortable—in this area, as they may see their roles as primarily curative. Dr. Mohs describes it as putting on a different hat. She believes it is an adjustment for a physician to switch from curative to palliative treatment:

> Sometimes, physicians who have collaborated with these people for 20-25 years consult us because they just can't make the switch. I felt that myself. It was harder for me to have those conversations with patients I have known for years. It is just more difficult. Not that an internist does not have those skills and cannot dance back and forth, but a lot of times, they don't, and so they don't develop that muscle that I think is unique to palliative care.

> But we live in a society where it's weird if you talk about death. It is weird to talk about death and to realize we are going to die and to approach that in any way but with fear or avoidance. I am trying to figure out how to present it and how to be with it so that it permeates the community and our nation without developing this culture of death. I think people really do feel creeped out by it.

As a neonatologist, Dr. Bair has been taking care of preemies and critically ill newborns for nearly 35 years. In his subset of medical practice, the care he provides is directed at the infant, but his relationship and communication skills are centered on the parents. The success of managing and extending the life of critically ill infants is what drew him into neonatology. But his career choice also meant delivering the news of an impending death to the parents of the most vulnerable of newborn babies. Dr. Bair's unique point of view confirms that the experience of loss is not diminished by the length of life. He has witnessed many different expressions of grief from his patient's families:

> I have seen the gamut. I have seen fathers literally lie down on the floor and beat on it. It is something to see a 300-pound man beating on the floor.

> We had one family where the dad literally came to pieces because he'd lost a set of twins on the same day in our unit, and then about a year and a half later, they lost a third child in our unit. The mother did much better than he did. He was literally beside himself.

> If you have been up on our floor there is a print of three cherubs, the framed cherubs. It was that family who had bought it as a remembrance of their kids. I cannot imagine. It goes back to what my grandmother said, a parent is not supposed to outlive their children.

Dr. Bair tells the story of a physician he trained under who was dubbed "the Grim Reaper." This physician would tell the family in a direct way that their baby would not survive. The news did not necessarily mean that treatment would stop at that moment, but it did provide the truth up front, as difficult as it could be to hear. For his part, Dr. Bair uses an analogy that helps him to convey to parents when their baby's life is no longer sustainable. He likens it to a ship and its rudder:

> You do get into a lot of issues where families just cannot accept it. And we basically find ourselves in a situation

where we've already approached the family because we know the baby is going to die. It is just a matter of waiting until it happens.

I will tell them, "I know you still want us to try everything; we are already telling you we have done everything."… Usually, by the time we get into a situation, and I am sure this [is the same with adult patients] too, if we have gotten to this point, it is because we can't reverse the underlying process. So, if the ship is still heading in that direction, I do not have a rudder. I cannot bring it back here. It is going to continue to travel in that direction no matter what I do. There is no point in trying to jump-start the motor when I have no rudder. So, we will take things like chest compressions and cardiac stimulants off the table. If the baby is not on a ventilator for some reason, we will explain that we are not going to intubate the baby and use a ventilator because that is not going to change this problem.

There are many ways patients can be informed that death is coming. Some are nuanced, but still make the message clear. Dr. Bair, received the blunt version in such a conversation with his father's physician after his father was diagnosed with multivalvular and inoperable congestive heart failure:

It was before the days of HIPPA, and I contacted his internist and asked, "Ok, what can we expect?"

He said, "I am guessing your dad has 1½ years to live."

I said, "Ok, does he know that?"

"No."

I said, "Are you going to tell him that?"

"No."

"Is there any particular reason you are not going to tell him that?"

He said, "I have had conversations with your dad [about] where he is in life. He is retired. He's got things in place. You kids are grown and out of the house, married, and have families. Your mother is financially ok from what your father has told me. My experience has been when I tell somebody that if they have 1½ years to live, they are going to sit on the edge of the couch and wait to die. What I did tell him was, 'Keith, are there things you want to do?' Your dad is smart; he read between the lines. I did not have to tell him that there is a time limit on this. It is a time-limited offer."

As it turned out my father lived three more years.

In other scenarios, physicians attempt to shield family members from the unwelcome news. This is a disservice to the family members who need to know the prognosis but are then left in the dark. Mary Catherine Wright shares her experience at age 19 with her mother's end-of-life story:

When my mom died, I was only 19. There were four of us kids. She had raised us by herself. I remember a nurse practitioner—this was in 1979, before there were a whole lot of advanced practice nurses. I remember they met with us kids twice because it was so traumatic for us. I remember that the doctor did not really talk to us, and I remember wondering why. The physician did not tell us about the cause of death or prognosis or meet with us. I think he was communicating with my Aunt Pat, my mom's sister. But I just remember thinking that this does not feel right. I could not really put it into words, but I am thinking that gosh, no one is talking to us. My mom had lung cancer. She smoked Pall Malls. I was only 19 and trying to get into nursing school and thinking that just did not seem right.

Then, it is funny, well, it is not funny. It's just that God has our paths, and years later, here I am talking to people and giving them a chance to ask questions and informing them and giving a listening ear.

There is a lot of satisfaction in knowing that you are helping people because I know what it was like trying to navigate blindly. We did not know. So, things have changed. I remember when we were not told anything and so it is very important to communicate, and I think the physician didn't really know how. It was too sorrowful for him to talk to four kids, Margaret's four children, so he communicated with my aunt. I would say it took me a good 20 years to work through the death of my mom.

Dr. Reitemeier believes that the use of words like "terminal wean," "brain death," and "poor prognosis" should not be used because people do not understand the meaning of these terms. Using vague language like this to convey that a patient is dying is an indication that even the healthcare team is uncomfortable talking about death. He urges care providers to be clear and transparent in their communication with families:

So, I will look them in the eye and ask, "Do you in your heart believe that that patient is going to die in that bed in that room?" When the physician responds, "Yes, that is what I believe," the family's reaction to that is "Really?" When the physician responds they have been trying to convey that for three weeks, my thought is that they have been failing at it for three weeks!

Stop using [vague] terms and stop looking for exit ramps. Do the hard work. Do not say "poor prognosis," say what you really believe. I do that at meetings, and I push the physician hard, and they hate it in the moment, and afterward, they say, "If you told me you were going to ask me that question in front of that family, I would have refused to go into the meeting. But you asked the question, I answered it, and that is what opened up everything."

Not all deaths are drawn out over time. There are unexpected deaths that take place from accidents, sudden heart attacks, COVID-19, and deaths by suicide. In these cases, loved ones may be spared what can feel like a tortuous and protracted goodbye, but they are also denied any opportunity to participate or assist their loved ones in closing the circle.

Whether a death occurs suddenly or at the end of a protracted dying process, those that are left behind are likely to experience a similar sense of deep loss and go through comparable periods of grief and mourning. But when a death occurs suddenly, or sometimes even when the family is able to grasp what is happening, the presence of unaddressed and unresolved family issues may cause family members and loved ones to struggle significantly more with the inevitable grief that comes to sit at the heart's doorstep. When death is recognized on the horizon and spoken about openly, it allows patients who are closing the circle the opportunity to express love, resolve disputes, and receive verification that their life had both meaning and meaningful relationships.

The role of fear

Blocking the idea of death or conversation about it may push back the grief that has started to surface, but it doesn't resolve the fear. Fear is the overlooked and unaddressed vital sign of healthcare. In fact, Dr. Reitemeier believes that the presence of fear can have a powerful influence on the delivery of end-of-life healthcare:

> We do not address fear because we do not know what to do with it. We cannot make it go away because it's legitimately there. Death is scary. And because we do not know how to make it go away, we do not even try to make it less.

Often, families are shocked when death occurs, even when there is a terminal or long-standing chronic illness. Family members can be taken by surprise because they may unwittingly further distance themselves from their loved one as death draws closer. Gail saw this phenomenon many times:

> I have seen family members, when they know their loved one is at the end of life, have trouble coming into the hospital room, standing close to the bed, or even touching them. I remember facilitating and taking time to help families approach their loved ones and also explaining to them about the medical environment. I would tell them what the machines were for and how the intravenous lines were giving medicines, fluids, and drugs to keep them comfortable. I would always ask them, "Does she look comfortable to you?"

The feeling of fear often associated with death can permeate thoughts, actions, and decision- making. Fear influences the patient, the family, and even the healthcare provider's ability to communicate. It shuts down the expression of emotion at a time when opening up is an important part of finding closure. Rev. Marshall observes:

> Often, we do not even use the word "dying" or "death." I teach the chaplains to use these words and try to get people to say them because it is a part of life.

> Along with it is the fear of dying. I have been with a lot of patients who will say things about being afraid, and they tell me, "I am dying." They will say things like, "I couldn't tell anybody else this." It is because the medical team is trying to be upbeat and encouraging, and the family wants them to smile and put forth their best and are saying everything is going to be ok. And all they really want to do is just kind of be afraid, be honest, scared, cry, and get it out. Then, when everyone else leaves the room and only

I am there, they might not verbalize it, but they will just start crying, and it will be followed by, "I am so afraid," "I could not tell my sister this," "I could not tell my brother this," or "I could not tell my mom this."

One of my pitches for spiritual support services is that we are people who can come along and just let people be real. They do not have to put up that brave front and fight to the end. That is fine. But even within my own family with people who say, "I'm tired of fighting, and I don't want to fight anymore; I'm done," they feel guilty. If they admit they are afraid, they feel guilty or shameful admitting it. We do not want to shame people. Let them be who they are. If they are feeling afraid, I tell them it is ok to be afraid. If they feel like giving in or just stopping treatment or quitting, that is ok.

Fear is a good coping mechanism for us. It helps us get through. Fear in and of itself is not necessarily a terrible thing. I just want people to experience where they are. Express where they are. If I can get a family to let their loved one express what they are feeling and their emotions, and we can all connect with that, typically they deal with fear better than when they try to repress it.

Rev. Marshall has seen how the acceptance of death can take various forms, and advises that healthcare providers must be attuned to the family for closure to take place:

One time, I was called to a room of a young man with many complications. He dwindled away, and he died. His mother had been in the room for hours, and she would not leave. The nurses sent for me to help.

It is one of those stories I really remember vividly. I walked in and sat down and just hung out with her for a while. She was speaking about, I forget his name, but she was speaking about "Bobby" as though Bobby was yet alive. That kind of freaked the nurses out because it had been several hours, and it was as if she did not realize it.

After I spent some time with her, I said, "Working here at the hospital, there are some things we have to do for your son Bobby, and I can't do them while you are here. We have had a wonderful time together, but at this point, I really need to do some things with him and for him that I can only do when you leave."

I was wondering and praying about how this was going to go over because I thought she was still saying there would be a miracle at any moment now. Then she said to me, "OK. If I leave, will he be cold, and will he be alone?" I said, "I promise you I will get another warm blanket, and if we remove him from this room, we will put him where there are some other people. He will not be alone."

She never said he was dead. Nor did I say it. She got up, and she kissed him, and I walked out with her and told the staff to do what you've got to do. I do not think I lied to her. I did get another blanket, and they took him to the morgue.

She was one of those who was, "I believe, I believe, I believe [he is not dead]," but she knew what had happened and she could accept it on her own terms in her own way. If we give it to them that way, it is easier.

Our fear of death and dying and our inability to manage that fear creates roadblocks to what could be a rich experience with those we love. Fear clouds our capacity to make rational decisions and cherish the last moments. The opportunity to close the circle with a good death is better realized when fear is acknowledged and addressed.

Anticipatory grief: Death's forerunner

When a patient or a family come to realize that death is the likely outcome, they can experience an emotion known as anticipatory grief. A person with anticipatory grief starts to experience sadness relating to how much life will change or how much a loved one will be missed. It is a common occurrence, but it can hinder clear thinking and the ability to make reasonable medical decisions. When anticipatory grief occurs, decisions that were agreed upon when death was not imminent suddenly become negotiable.

Joanne Lax, JD, was a pivotal addition to the clinical ethics committee. She specialized in healthcare law and was awarded Best Lawyer in Healthcare in Detroit in 2012. During case reviews, she was a valuable contributor to the consultation team's work, keeping track of the case's ethical issues with compassion and insight. Her experience with how her father reversed his previously expressed wishes during a serious illness is a prime example of how anticipatory grief can affect decision-making:

> My dad had all kinds of peripheral vascular disease and heart disease. He ended up with one amputation and went into a nursing home and was just absolutely miserable in the nursing home.
>
> He was fully competent, but he had become a huge curmudgeon because he could not do things for himself that he wanted to do and he did not want to be there, and on and on and on. He told us, "If ever they say I need another amputation, I am not having it. Even if they say I am going to die, I am not having it." Well, the day came when they said he needed a second amputation. And my mother was there talking to him, and the next thing I knew, he was going to surgery for the second amputation.
>
> I thought, *holy cow, if I had been his surrogate, I would have made exactly the opposite decision.* But the two of them,

together, were talking about the current situation, and I do not know what she said to him. It was all a private conversation. I think it was something along the lines of, "I cannot stand the thought of you not being here, Erv. I will always be here in the nursing home with you, and I will take care of you, and I will be your angel here, whatever you want." And [he decided] that is what he wanted. He was equally miserable after the second amputation.

Joanne's mother's anticipatory grief drove her father to go back on what he originally wanted.

Anticipatory grief's emotional pain comes in part from the looming sense of loss that it creates—not only the loss of a person, but also the loss of a dream. Neonatologist Dr. Bair experienced something akin to this firsthand:

My son was diagnosed with autism at age three. That was so long ago that we knew nothing about autism. I mean, literally, I could pull out a pediatric text and find one paragraph on autism out of hundreds and hundreds of pages. That is how little we knew about it at the time.

I did not want to hear that my son had autism, and we went through that same feeling with our families (who also did not want to hear unwelcome news). Although my son never died, he is as healthy as a horse, I understood emotionally what they are going through because I understand death. My dream died. It was the idea that I would have a son that would go on to marry, have a family, which is gone. It still makes me cry. And you could not ask for a nicer young man who was more talented. So, I certainly have a soft spot and feel for families that are going through this. But I still have a child at the end of the day, and they do not.

Dr. Bair recounts a particular case that involved a full-term baby that looked perfect but had a complex oxygenation problem, causing almost immediate death after birth. This case of anticipatory grief included the loss of an imagined future:

> It still makes me cry to think about it. I can deal with a woman crying. I am married. But to see a grown man cry, you do not see that very often. What made it really hard was that it was a term baby, a big, fat, chubby baby. The dad is sitting there, and we are both staring at this beautiful cherub that is dying, literally. The nurses are crying, the dad's crying, the mom is not there. She is back in L and D. It was right after birth. We moved the baby back there immediately. What got me was the father was going through the list of things he would never get to do with his daughter. Many of those I had already done with mine. I just sat there and held him for a while, but then I thought it was inappropriate for me to sit here and bawl, so I left him and went to my call room and bawled. Then I came home and hugged my kids. That was probably 23 years ago.

This father's grief existed not only for his child in that moment, but also in anticipation of the many losses he would again experience in the future.

Anticipatory grief can result in compromised decision-making by family members who realize how the death of a loved one will also change their own lives. There are accounts relating to this phenomenon in previous chapters. In Chapter 3, Gail observed how Charlie's wife's anticipatory grief over losing her husband was complicated by the fact she was dependent on his income to survive. Eileen Dunleavy discussed how she has witnessed many adult sons who live with and are supported by a parent, and how they are not equipped to have their own lives upended by that parent's death. In these and similar cases, the family member grapples with both the loss of their loved one and the life that they know. It is anticipatory grief that often prompts a family to ask their dying loved one to "fight on," and in turn, the patient tries to do so to grant his partner or children extra time.

When death is on the horizon, fear and anticipatory grief are important emotions for the healthcare provider to recognize not only in family members, but in patients, too. Sometimes, a patient's wish for continued treatment arises from a desire to resolve conflicts and a fear there won't be enough time for them to be resolved. Dr. Reitemeier's previous story about the patient who begged her physician to keep her alive long enough for her children to gather together and make peace with each other is an example of this. Her grief about ongoing discord between those she loved hindered her acceptance of death, the closing of her circle.

The ability to identify and acknowledge fear and anticipatory grief may make the difference between a good, bad, or ugly death. Martha believes that it is helpful for healthcare providers to recognize how death's ripple effect may be impacting family members' behavior:

> At some point during my experience in supporting families, I came to understand that there is no such thing as the death of a single person. Death is happening to everyone in the family, to all loved ones. The grief that families experience is generated not only because of the impending loss of the patient, but also a feeling of a loss of one's self. There is inclusiveness to dying. Maybe that is why some loved ones hold on so hard when they really should be letting go.

For the healthcare providers it is important to understand not only the emotional but also the physical effects of anticipatory grief on patients and their loved ones. In "Grief Counseling and Grief Therapy," W. Worden (2018) describes the physical manifestations of normal grieving. These symptoms include hollowness in the stomach, tightness in the chest, tightness in the throat, oversensitivity to noise, a sense of depersonalization, breathlessness, feeling short of breath, weakness in the muscles, lack of energy, and dry mouth. Physical symptoms such as these can also compromise comprehension and decision-making, just as anticipatory grief's psychological impacts can.

Anticipatory grief is a complex phenomenon with a variety of outcomes. Father Leliaert taught a class about death and dying for 10 years at Nazareth College in Kalamazoo, Michigan. He also worked in England under the oversight of social worker Dr. Susan Le Poidevin, who was well known for her work in grief support. During his time there he learned about the surprising benefit of anticipatory grief:

> In England, it was a "stiff upper lip," and I experienced that. Talk about cultural stuff. I did enough work to really get a feel for good old English grief.

> Susan began to work with me in her model of working through grief. She trusted me enough to send me to various places in England to speak…to people who wanted to know more about death and dying.

> [There is a value to] engaging in the grieving processes quite a while before death. You did not take away, necessarily, the pain, but it would help to alleviate the full impact so that after the death, the person's grief process would take on a more life-giving form.

> Some people hold on to the very end and afterwards they cannot shake it because they are so involved in grief that sometimes 10 years later, they never really get their life back. So anticipatory grief became very important to me. I found it extremely helpful in my own practice, both as an educator and eventually as a chaplain and a priest in the healthcare setting.

Both universal and unique

Chris Westphal's analogy for dealing with end-of-life as a healthcare provider captures the uniqueness of the experience. She believes that working with patients who are closing the circle is like dancing with a partner. You adjust and maneuver together depending on changing circumstances. It requires give and take, reading the signs, and discovering the steps that will give this moment meaning and cohesion. Helping someone who is dying means allowing the expression of fear. It also requires understanding that a patient's or family's acceptance of death can have many pathways.

In many cases and for most families, once these elements were granted recognition, acceptance of death became possible. This was especially true when discussions already occurred prior to a crisis, or when a patient had clearly expressed their wishes about the sort of existence that would be acceptable to them. Whether it was in conversation or in the form of an advance medical directive, having an awareness of a patient's wishes paved an easier path for closing the circle. And though grief will be present, it is not as likely exacerbated by doubt, anxiety or guilt.

For Gail and those who traveled in her orbit of accumulated knowledge and compassion, the path to a good death began first with a respect for the wishes of the patient, followed by empathy, trust, and open communication and education. Because in the end, a good death is more likely to occur when open communication and acceptance are used to manage grief and fear.

Join our Circle

- Gail said, "Being able to talk with someone about death [can be difficult] because it is hard to deal with your own mortality." **How do your thoughts and feelings about your own death impact the conversations you have with patients and families about end of life? How do you manage those thoughts and feelings when you are providing end-of-life care?**

- Dr. Hnatiuk observed that many physicians are uncomfortable discussing death because they have not had any formal training in how to talk to a patient or their family about death and dying. **Have you ever had any instruction in how to talk to patients and families about death? What kind of training do you think would be most helpful for healthcare providers in addressing this subject?**

- When Dr. Bair needed to inform the parents of his neonatal patients that their baby's life was no longer sustainable, he used the metaphor of a ship and rudder. **Have you discovered or observed an effective way of delivering difficult messages such as this so that families can understand and absorb it?**

- Dr. Reitmeier urges healthcare providers to communicate clearly and avoid formal medical jargon when communicating about death: "Stop using those terms and stop looking for exit ramps. Do the hard work. Do not say 'poor prognosis'; say what you really believe." **Can you recall a time when you caught yourself communicating with a patient or family member in a way that reflected your discomfort with the conversation? How do you make yourself "do the hard work"?**

- When Gail was working in critical care units, she tried to alleviate family members' fear by taking the time to help them approach their loved ones and explaining the medical equipment that surrounded them. **How do you help patients and families work through their fear around death and dying?**

- Anticipatory grief is a common occurrence, but it can hinder clear thinking and the ability to make reasonable medical decisions. **Have you experienced or observed anticipatory grief in a hospital environment? What are some ways to address and mitigate some of the negative effects it may have?**

Chapter 6

Understanding the Connection: Communicating with Patients and Family

Studies have shown that family members with loved ones in the ICU rate communication with their healthcare providers as one of the most important skills for these providers. In fact, most families rate the clinician's communication skills, along with the continuity and accessibility, as more important than their clinical skills.

Curtis et al.

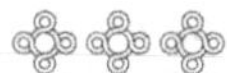

We've addressed the value of good communication in the hospital setting, but here we are dedicating an entire chapter to this topic because its importance cannot be overstated, especially in your interactions with patients and families who are going through end-of-life experiences. Good communication skills allow you to build the trust, understanding, and support that are necessary for patients to achieve a good death.

Gail encouraged Family Matters staff to pay special attention to the way they communicated with patients and families, and she supported and advised them when they encountered tough communication scenarios on the job.

While our colleagues brought a variety of backgrounds and perspectives to the table, they all stressed that empathy is an essential communication skill during challenging interactions with stressed and anxious patients and family members. In this chapter, we share some of their experiences and the philosophical and practical lessons that they offer for effective communication in healthcare settings.

Communication is so important to the patient experience that hospital systems ask patients to rate their satisfaction with staff communication in their discharge surveys. Every level of healthcare education should include training for enhancing communication between the provider and the patient.

In the hospital setting, skillful communication requires both relaying healthcare information and being attuned to the emotional impact the information may have on the recipients. Throughout her career, Gail developed strategies for healthcare providers to communicate effectively:

> It is important to recognize there is a process to good communication and establishing a relationship of trust.
>
> First, it's important to engage the patient or family, to get their attention and convey to them that your role is to help them understand the complexities of what they may be facing. You need to use terms that are understandable to them, and to recognize that their understanding or acceptance may come in degrees. You need to be accessible to them and let them know how they can contact you.
>
> Sometimes there is a need to address language barriers or misunderstandings based on different cultural interpretations. Sometimes you find that among the family members there are different motives and agendas.
>
> Each case is different. Often people are overwhelmed and not processing what they are being told.

Gail was keenly aware of how the stressful events like a life-threatening heart attack or the diagnosis of a debilitating long-term chronic illness affected patients' and families' ability to comprehend what was happening.

Stress, illness, and comprehension

In initial conversations with healthcare providers, patients and families want to find out what is wrong (the diagnosis) and what can be done to correct it (the treatment options). But if it becomes evident that a condition is serious, emotions such as fear and anxiety begin to surface. Faced with the possibility of a decline in physical or mental ability or even death, the patient and family's previous assumptions about what their future holds begin to disintegrate. In the emotional upheaval that accompanies this news, information given by the provider often goes unheard.

Because they lose focus on what is being said, patients and families often request that providers repeat information, or they fail to comprehend what they are being told—circumstances that are often misconstrued by the healthcare team as inattentiveness.

So, at a time when a clear head is crucial for decision-making, stress can disrupt the ability to retain and process information.

Gail and the Family Matters staff encountered many situations in which the family members claimed they had not been updated or informed of the patient's status. Gail remembers:

> It was not unusual for family members in the ICU to ask for an update about what was happening with a loved one. There were many occasions in which the physician would meet with the patient and family members and provide the latest news regarding the plan of care and the current condition. But often, even during the same day, we would be approached by family who expressed that they did not know what was going on and asked for someone to "talk to us." This resulted in physicians expressing frustration that they had just done that, and had answered all their questions.

Learning what worked: Techniques for effective communication

Healthcare providers should view these behaviors as an opportunity to re-evaluate how they are providing information. One way to gauge whether a message is being understood is to begin by asking the patient and family what they think is happening. Then, the providers deliver information in short, understandable terms and ask the listener to repeat it. This technique, known as an Ask-Tell-Ask feedback model,[1] is a useful tool in the healthcare setting. When the healthcare provider engages in a back-and-forth dialogue with the family, it allows time for comprehension. It also serves as a litmus test to help healthcare providers recognize when to reframe when the information is not understood.

Gail and Family Matters staff also used another technique to communicate effectively with anxious patients and families:

> We were asked by an intensivist to develop a "family meeting" form. The form included a place to record the time, date, and duration of the meeting, who attended, the purpose of the meeting, the issues discussed, and the next steps or plan of care. A family member was given a copy of the completed form, and a copy was also placed in the medical record.

> It was a device to capture the information the patient or family may not have been able to process during the meeting itself. It was not that the patient or family were not trying to understand the facts, [it's that] they were also trying to make sense of what the information would mean for them, how life would change.

Family members would often refer to the form because stress and

---

1   *For more information on this topic, please see the Resources section at the end of the book.*

worry about their loved one's condition affected their memory of the conversation. This document was not only helpful to the family, but to the other healthcare providers because it provided an account of what had already been discussed.

While a healthcare provider may be experienced in delivering bad news, the patient is nevertheless receiving this news for the first time. Ethicist Dr. Reitemeier was often consulted on cases where physicians encountered an impasse in a patient or family's understanding of how dire a situation was, and the unlikelihood of successful treatment. He stresses that when relaying life-altering news, not only the word choice but also the timing and pacing of information is important:

> There is a difference between the message and the package that it is delivered in. You have the message, but you screw up the packaging. Not everything has to be given in the same conversation. Not everything has to be given in the same sentence.

> So, get your words right because it's going to be repeated. If you do it awkwardly and brutally it is going to be amplified awkwardly and brutally. If you do it gently, slowly, and softly, that will be carried forward as well.

> And remember that as soon as the word "cancer" is used by the physician, or "malignancy" or any other well understood synonym for cancer, nothing else can be heard that day.

Dr. Reitemeier used a consistent process to communicate with stressed family members:

> I always start every meeting with family members with the same three questions:

> "Why is your dad in the hospital?" [Then] I see what they answer to [that question].

Second question: "What are the nurses and doctors doing for him?" "Doing" is a very important verb because it's wide open.

And the third question is: "In your opinion, how well is it working?"

Dr. Reitemeier also remarked that healthcare providers never fail to be surprised at how little the family truly understands what is happening even after hours of conversations about a patient's diagnosis. Not only do patients and families fail to understand what they are being told, but they can also misinterpret information.

"You have wasted hours of repeating medicalese," he explained. "You might as well have been speaking Thai. But they are too polite to say, 'I don't get it. Try again.'"

The primary goal of Family Matters staff was to optimize communication. FMSS staff members invested time and energy in facilitating communication, meeting family members at the bedside or in waiting rooms and making phone calls across the country and even internationally. Each day staff would review the medical record, speak with the care providers, conduct a bedside visit, and field calls from family. There were times when conveying information involved calling prison inmates, using interpreters, or organizing numerous family meetings.

But Family Matters staff did not just assist with communication logistics. The FMSS approach to patients and families, developed by Gail and Chris Westphal, centered on patient self-determination, inclusion of family, truth-telling, and culturally congruent care. This approach prepared staff to contribute to sensitive discussions that involved everything from who should be a spokesperson to withdrawing life support. They became skilled in judging how information should be delivered and recognizing when extra support was needed.

As Family Matters grew more established, its staff continued to develop techniques to communicate more effectively. Chris, with her combination of experience in Family Matters, critical care, and palliative care, strongly advocated scheduling a family meeting by the third day of a patient's stay in the critical care unit. Superior to the typical quick hallway updates, a scheduled meeting provides families with information, answers their questions, and determines next steps. It is an opportunity for the available consulting physicians to explain the patient's medical status to the family, as well as review the patient's expressed wishes. Chris described best practices for these family meetings:

> The family needs to be informed of what day and time the meeting will be held and requested that they arrange their schedules. The family then needs to be told that in the meeting they will be informed if the patient is progressing and if the goal of care is on track. A second meeting should then be scheduled again on day six or sooner if the condition changes.

In addition to scheduling consistent meetings in advance, Chris found that providing a meeting summary was also highly beneficial for communication and transparency, both essential factors in effective medical decision-making.

With her nursing experience in the ICU and as a consultant in ethics, Eileen Dunleavy participated in countless patient and family conversations. Whether doing bedside care or participating in an ethics consultation, her initial goal was to establish rapport and build relationships. In addition to this, Eileen learned to gather as much information as possible from key participants and then record the interactions through chart notes:

> When I get an ethics consult, the first thing I do is review the chart, including the reason for the consult. I then call the person who ordered the consult to get a

better understanding of the ethical tensions in the case. I always make a bedside visit to lay eyes on the patient and introduce myself and my role if the patient is able to interact. I attempt to speak with all stakeholders, including the bedside nurse who often has the most complete information outside the chart. I document all this in the chart. I then continue with my next steps in formulating an analysis.

Unfortunately, healthcare providers are often caught in a continuous cycle of "rediscovering" information that someone else had already learned but did not record, or that was not reviewed by other healthcare team members. This is especially true of cases involving a large family or many medical consultants. Properly recording information not only benefits the healthcare team, but it also relieves the family from being continually bombarded with the same questions.

Eileen used this method when she relayed medical information:

> When I am talking with the patient or family, I do not have a problem with telling them about medical issues because I am taking information out of the chart and relaying it to them. It's not like I am interjecting any opinion. I think it helps when they see the picture laid out for them. Communication is key. If you just meet and make contact and put all the pieces together with them, sometimes the puzzle just falls into place, and they can see what is happening.

The analogy of putting together a puzzle is very appropriate. It conveys that information delivered in smaller pieces and at the right pace allows the patient and family to comprehend the big picture. This approach often creates an opportunity for an "aha" moment that clarifies the decisions that need to be made.

Good communication in a medical setting should be deliberate, clear, and methodical, but Family Matters staff also found that it could be personal and empathetic. Mary Catherine Wright has worked in many healthcare settings: parish nursing, Family Matters, hospice, and nursing home administration. In all of these settings, she drew from her personal experiences to communicate with patients and build relationships with them:

> I remember Gail would talk about finding our commonality with others, and I had done that, I guess subconsciously, when I was doing parish nursing. I did not really have any formal training, but it just was a natural fit for me. I had experienced a lot of death and end-of-life issues in my own personal life. My mom had died when I was only 19. My Aunt Pat, who was my mentor, died. My grandparents and uncles had died. So, I was dealing with death on a personal level and trying to make sense of all that. So, it just seemed like a nice fit [when I was] talking to people…that I could relate to them. I could relate to them and their sorrow and try to get through it.

> There were some similarities with [working with the community in parish nursing and] working in acute care. People are people, and you try to find the commonality… People also just want to be listened to. In the community they wanted me to listen, if it was in their front room or in their kitchen, and at the hospital they wanted me to listen to them. Those were the similarities.

A healthcare provider's responsibility

When Dr. Mohs read the book *Crucial Conversations: Tools for Talking When Stakes Are High* (Patterson et al., 2012), she came to appreciate the "high stakes" nature of communication in the hospital setting and better understand the fight-or-flight reaction people experience when conversations feel threatening, or when there is a high risk of loss.

Dr. Mohs stressed how important good communication skills are at these times:

> Basically, the stakes are always high in the hospital. The stakes are high for administration, the stakes are high for nurses, the stakes are high for therapists, and ancillary services, physicians, and the stakes are high for the patients, the family. There is never a time when the stakes are not high. It's when the stakes are high that you are most likely to get in a situation where you are going to get in a crucial conversation…

> If you don't know how to handle them as a crucial conversation, if you don't recognize it, you can get into a fight, frankly. You can just totally blow it…

> So when we get into that situation where the stakes are high and there may be a difference of opinion and good communication is required, or our hearts are beating fast and maybe we are a little bit afraid, we know that this is important and our natural instinct is to fight or fly.

> I think there is that crucial conversation element of it that I've now come to appreciate is a skill. That is part of what palliative care [providers] must be able to do, is to have those kinds of conversations. To be able to greet that [emotion], no matter how it comes out, whether it comes out in tears, whether it comes out [they] have suspicions, whether it comes out they have anger, whether it comes out [as] fear. You have to be able to stand there and navigate that because you're the one who knows what's happening right now. Both in terms of a diagnostician and as a person [who] is not in it…

> As a professional I need to come to that table and be the one who keeps things moving in the right direction in terms of communication. I need to be skilled in conversation because I cannot depend on them to be

skilled, even when they are skilled, because it's a tough situation [and] they are in it.

Dr. Mohs calls on healthcare providers to be aware of how adept or lacking their own skills are in communicating information, especially life-changing information, because she believes that communicating well is the professional's responsibility. She attributes the development of her own communication skills to Gail's guidance and her experience as co-chair of the System Clinical Ethics Committee with Dr. Weber. Similar to her experience in palliative care, Dr. Mohs's experience in clinical ethics solidified her desire to work with people who were going through the most challenging times of their lives, which gave her many opportunities to help others navigate when their stakes are high.

Though he is a skilled communicator in multiple languages, Mohamad (Moe) Rustom also encountered the challenges and boundaries of patient communication in his roles as a registered nurse, clinical ethics and Family Matters staff, and Director of Clinical Interpretation and Translation Services:

> I always understood my part to be a communicator and to explain things. I cannot give someone else the courage to decide what to do, but I have always tried to make it as easy as possible for him or her to comprehend the consequences. I spent a lot of time educating people, telling them stories, and explaining what they may not understand. Remember, you are not talking to medical people; you are talking to people who might be seeing a ventilator for the first time. You must explain all of that.
>
> I was inclusive and I communicated and educated. I am very proud of the role I played, but I did not see myself persuading people in a direction to make a specific decision. But I did know that they needed to understand everything. Even with limited knowledge people need to understand

everything to make the right decision to suit their own needs and suit their view of life and death, not mine.

I would explain to our recent immigrant Muslim patients the reason why the doctor would come in and tell them what is happening was because in this country we have laws that give people the right to know. Patients or families from another ethnicity or religion might ask, "Why is the doctor telling me that?" In some cultures, the healthcare provider doesn't even talk to you. It happened to me when I went home to see my hospitalized mother in Lebanon.

I tried to empower people with understanding through communication. Communication is key, key, to everything. People need to know. Yet the struggle to make the decision is not yours or mine. The struggle is theirs.

Moe found himself having to apply what he learned about patient communication in his own life:

First you need to explain everything about the situation and consider how it will be received. It is what I did for my brothers and sister. I told them about our mother's cancer and the effects it had on her body. I told them I had never heard of a case like hers where someone survived. You must build toward a level of understanding and then let them make the decision. I did make the decision for my family, but I still had to get their consensus and we all agreed.

For Moe, successful communication was about clearly transferring information without bias or opinion, and avoiding assumptions about how the patient or family would act upon the information given to them. For example, if the healthcare provider walks into a family meeting with the intention of making the patient a "no code," but the patient or family is not aware of a poor prognosis or is not emotionally ready to limit care, it is not surprising when they refuse. Obtaining informed consent to not resuscitate may seem reasonable to the provider, but what is primarily important is to communicate the pros and cons of resuscitation and how it may affect quality of life. Then the patient or family is allowed to decide the course of action, whatever it may be. This point was articulated by ethicist Dr. Weber:

> There was a tendency on the part of some physicians, not all by any means, to be paternalistic. You cannot have informed consent if you're deciding for somebody else what's the right thing to do, and that's what paternalism means. But you have to be able to tell the true story to the best of your ability, even if the true story is "We don't know."

> That's fine, but to tell that. And so, the ability to tell that is not easy for a lot of physicians. The nature of the workload makes it even more difficult because they are not always available when the people are available to talk. This is how ethics consults can facilitate informed consent because they can say, "Everyone take a break from what you're doing and come together in this little conference room here. This is what we have to talk about."

> But you have to be there and provide your medical understanding of what the condition is, what the expectations are going down the line, what you can do in terms of treatment, what you cannot do in terms of treatment. You provide all that so that [the patient or family] can then make an informed decision based upon *their* understanding of what is valuable and important to *them*, about whether that's acceptable or not.

It's important to note that in this scenario, the provider proposes limiting care and allows the patient or family to make that decision. This situation is different from a case in which the healthcare provider makes that determination alone based on the certainty that resuscitation will be non-beneficial. In that case, it is not a subjective judgment, an opinion about "quality of life," but rather a medical determination based on best practice. And although the patient or family may not be part of the decision-making in those circumstances, they must still be informed about it.

Both Moe and Dr. Weber's accounts take into consideration not only communication methods, but also communication challenges. Healthcare providers are challenged by lack of time, lack of training in communication skills, cultural misconceptions, and their own personal attitudes and reservations about conveying bad news. Even the most adept communicators in the Family Matters community faced and learned from the variety of different challenges they encountered.

Dr. Reitemeier understands the difficulties that healthcare providers face when unwelcome news needs to be delivered, but he challenges the belief that patients or family members do not want to be told unwelcome news. As was mentioned in Chapter 2 on trust and truth-telling, he has a different interpretation of people's resistance to hearing the truth: "They desperately want to know. They just don't want it to be true."

The communication challenge here is multifaceted. The healthcare provider has information they know will be devastating and life-changing for the family to hear, and yet the provider must determine when and how to convey it. When a patient or family hears unwelcome news, it can trigger a variety of emotions, such as fear, denial, or grief. A patient's or family's reaction may be a wild card, but the unpredictability of their reaction shouldn't compromise the principles of good communication. During these conversations, the challenge for healthcare providers is to be both the communicator of information and the recipient of family reactions, whatever they may be.

Mary Catherine learned a method of coping with adverse reactions from Gail:

Some people talk by yelling. I remember Gail would tell me that we had to put on our "brass brassiere." Sometimes I would use that phrase and people I worked with would ask, "What is she talking about?" But I realized what that was. I had to be tough. I had to be ready to handle the way a person was trying to communicate.

People who are skilled at relaying news to family can be an important asset when communication is critical. Rev. Marshall explains that as the hospital chaplain he was sometimes asked to intercede on the part of the medical team to help them get the message across so the family would see an inevitable outcome:

> There have been multiple times when families just do not hear and understand what has been told to them. I will sit there listening, and the medical team may leave and ask me why they do not get it. I try to rephrase things and do it from other perspectives and ask the family to express what they have heard. Then I can go back to the physician and say, "I know what you said but this is what they heard and I don't think these are the same two things. Let's try again."

> And when the family trusts you, and we use that to our benefit—when they see me as Reverend, and they trust the Reverend—then I am going to use that to help the family. I can come along and be a friend if they trust me. I have had to have some of those difficult conversations and to say point blank, "There is nothing else the medical team can do, we are at that point, and this is the end. We put your loved one in the hands of God. We are people of faith. I have seen God do what I think are miracles and I have also seen the miracle of God calling a loved one home. This is where we are. Let us trust in God."

This sentiment, the need to trust and connect, is commonly seen as essential for successful communication among healthcare providers. Serious illness exposes our mortality and makes us feel vulnerable. But, once the possibility of dying emerges, the human need to connect becomes stronger. This creates an opportunity for healthcare providers to connect through attentiveness and the words we use.

The connection between the healthcare provider and patient can be nurtured with simple measures such as active listening, acknowledging family ties, answering questions, and being open and receptive to thoughts, feelings, and needs. These tactics can be employed even during brief encounters. More important than the length of the interaction is the sincerity and focus the healthcare provider shows.

Even when using these techniques, sometimes achieving a rapport with a patient is challenging. However, these situations can provide a better understanding of your communication strengths and weaknesses. Dr. Mohs remembers a patient who communicated with her through consistent hostility and expressions of anger:

> I remember sitting there and trying to talk to him and engage him in conversation and it was like he was trying to piss me off. And he actually did. I was mad and told him there's more to me than what he was making me out to be. I finally got mad at him…and he relaxed. He basically told me, "Now you're real. Now it's real." And I thought it was interesting.

> It had an impact on me, and I became aware of how often I can put up that guard and not really be present. It can almost be condescending if you aren't present, if you feel like you have to separate, if you feel like you have to put up that demeanor and always stay reasonable and in control. It can be perceived as condescending.

> I think that the cases that impact me the most are those when I see someone who is kind of stuck in anger or stuck

in denial or stuck somewhere in that grieving process and then transitions. It is when you know they are grieving, you know that this is deep grief and then they are able to move past it, at least for now. Or you see a different facet of what they are actually going through. When that happens it's definitely poignant and impacts me. I think of particular cases and for some reason it is mostly anger, or anger that transitions to connection. For some reason that seems to be a common theme.

Healthcare providers may face many challenges in communicating effectively with patients and families. During critical illness or end-of-life experiences, patients and families are likely to feel difficult emotions like fear, grief, and anger, leading them to resist a healthcare provider's attempts at communication or struggle to comprehend them. In addition to this, differences in culture, family dynamics, spirituality, education, age, and other factors may also result in communication obstacles between patient and provider. However, healthcare providers must face and overcome these obstacles to achieve the clarity necessary for patients and families to make informed medical decisions.

Communication and closing the circle

Ideally, when communication is open and transparent among the patient, the family, and the healthcare team, healthcare providers can better assist the patient closing the circle on their own terms. When the patient and family begin to discuss how to find closure, they sometimes express special needs or requests. For Family Matters staff, this could result in coordinating with spiritual support or social work services. It could also involve gifting a donated handmade blanket or arranging transcontinental calls or video calls. Some of the more memorable closure requests

FMSS staff helped arrange included P.A.W.S., our pet visitation program; a wedding and reception for a dying patient and their longtime partner in the ICU; a full-body-immersion baptism for a patient on a ventilator; and coloring the hair of a comatose patient at end of life after her daughters told staff their mother would be horrified that her white roots were visible. Music was another common request, and it was often beautifully sung at the bedside by Chaplain Beverly Beltramo.

While open communication often resulted in these beautiful moments, sometimes healthcare providers are unable to establish trust. Sometimes a fracture in the family interferes with decision-making and is not resolvable. Sometimes grief and fear drown out the information that is being communicated. It was not always a perfect ending, but what seemed to be key to helping the patient and family achieve a meaningful end-of-life experience is the healthcare provider's willingness to, as Rev. Marshall said, "walk along with families" and allow the process to take the provider to the place it needed to go. Sometimes those places were surprising to him:

> I hope my students understand that what I have learned is that I do not have the answers. Recognizing that I do not have the answers helps me to find how to connect with people. If I, or anyone, goes into the situation thinking, *I know what this family needs, I know what this is like,* I think that is dangerous ground. You are imposing something on them that may not be there. Even if you understand the family dynamics and all of that you will be surprised at how often people may go another way on us, a whole other place, and we will miss it. So do not always go by the nods and the smiles but really get the person to express where they are. That would be more of a teachable thing.

> Such a place came for me when a patient had died and he had young adults, late teens, maybe early-20s children,

and they were responding kind of funny to his death. I remember pulling them aside. I just wanted to know where they were. They were kind of testing me without really saying too much. Then one of them said something like, "I'm glad the SOB is dead," and he got ready to leave.

I was not shocked. I could have said, "Oh my!" There was a part of me that was thinking, *Ooh, really?* But then I started to think, *Now I am cracking the surface. They are inviting me in a little bit.* So, I said, "Really? Tell me about it. What is that about? It sounds like you have some emotions. What are they?"

They were angry. It turned out that he was a horrible father, abusive. They had every right to be glad he was dead but who were they going to say that to? How deep are those family secrets? They aren't going to get up at the funeral and say, "I'm glad the SOB is dead."

So that is anger and emotion that they are probably going to sit on. I allowed them to go back in the room. We shut the door [and I said] "Tell him now."

They cursed him out and said things they could not say when he was alive. When they expressed those horrible things, they became very emotional. They cried a lot. They got a little loud, and I was a little worried. I was like, *Okay, can people hear this?*

But I think they were better for it. Why? Because I created a safe place for them to be just where they were and from there, we could do work together. Had I just simply said a prayer and said, "Bless you all. You miss your dad. I know your dad loved you."…Well, I do not know that. I cannot make those statements. So that is the advice I try to give my students and that I live with when dealing with families and patients.

Rev. Marshall's account shows that closing the circle may not be the same for everyone. It also highlights that not only the patient, but also the family has a need to find closure, a meaning or understanding of how the life and death of someone else affected their own life. No matter what path it takes, it can be a remarkable experience and privilege to witness. When Family Matters staff gave recognition to the patient as a person and to the relationships that were vital to them, it revealed many times over that the role of a healthcare provider at end of life is creative, interactive, and a profoundly intimate glimpse at life's closing moments. In each instance, communication was key, requiring talking and listening, empathy and compassion, and creating relationships through dialogue.

Join our Circle

- Healthcare providers often use the Ask-Tell-Ask feedback model to determine if patients and families have understood the information the provider is giving them. This is particularly important when they are delivering the life-altering news of a serious or debilitating diagnosis. **What techniques do you use to check if patients and families are hearing and understanding what you are telling them?**

- When she was working in the critical care unit, Chris Westphal found it helpful to schedule a formal family meeting to provide information, answer questions, and determine next steps. Staff documented these meetings and provided families with a written summary of who attended, what was discussed, and any decisions that were made. **What best practices do you follow to make sure that communication with families is organized and transparent?**

- Eileen Dunleavy made sure to record as much information as possible in the chart notes. This helped prevent the "cycle of rediscovering," where healthcare providers spend time finding out information that someone else had already learned but did not record. **What methods do you find useful to capture all the relevant information related to a patient's treatment?**

- Regarding her experience having "crucial conversations" with patients and families, Dr. Mohs said, "I need to be skilled in conversation because I cannot depend on them to be skilled." **What conversational skills do you think are most important for good communication with patients and families?**

- Even with practice and experience, sometimes achieving a rapport with a patient is challenging. However, this can provide a better understanding of your communication strengths and weaknesses. **What are your greatest strengths as a communicator? What areas or skills would you like to improve on in your communication with patients and families?**

Advance Directives

Use your voice…before you lose your choice.

—Thomas Condon

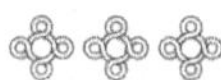

While there are many ways to communicate effectively about closing the circle, in this chapter we will discuss one of the most powerful: advance directives.

An advance medical directive is a legal document that records a person's preferences for the medical care they would want to receive if they become incapacitated and are unable to speak for themselves. It also designates someone the person trusts to ensure that their wishes are carried out.

Gail and her colleagues saw many times over how the presence of an advance directive made the difference between a good death and a bad or ugly one. Because of this, she created the advance directive document My Voice - My Choice, a labor of love that reflects the many lessons she and her colleagues learned about the end-of-life experience. This achievement represents the heart of Gail's work and the pinnacle of what she strove for throughout her career: truth-telling, education, informed decision-making, and honoring a person's right to choose.

We hope that this chapter will help you grow more familiar with these important documents, not just so you can educate your patients about them, but also so that they can inspire you to reflect on and communicate your wishes about your own end-of-life care.

A person's right to make decisions for themselves is based on the principles of autonomy and self-determination. Gail's steadfast belief in those principles led to one of her great successes: the creation of an exemplary advance directive document, *My Voice - My Choice* (MVMC).[2] Her efforts were spurred by the countless times she witnessed how important it was to have prior knowledge of patients' wishes for their end-of-life experience, and how that knowledge contributed to the challenges, heartbreaks, or peaceful resolutions of closing the circle:

> Everything that we did in developing *My Voice - My Choice* had to do with real life experiences and how to make the conversation happen and to find out what was important to the person. What medical treatment they would want or not want.

Capturing end-of-life wishes became of paramount importance to Gail. To communicate this issue's importance to others, she created the MVMC document and then zealously educated staff, patients and the community about it.

The history of advance directives

In the 1960s and 70s, medical technology accelerated. Its increasing sophistication, along with skyrocketing medical costs, resulted in the ability to sustain and prolong life by artificial means. This technological revolution coincided with a shift in the paradigm of medical decision-making from paternalism to autonomy. The first legal statute to support this shift was introduced in California in 1976 and was referred to as a "living will."

Several landmark court cases brought to light the importance of having a document to respect a person's medical choices. One

---

2   *For more information on My Voice - My Choice, please see the Resources section at the end of the book.*

famous case was that of Nancy Cruzan,[3] a young single woman who had a car accident in 1983 that left her in a persistent vegetative state. After years of Nancy being fed through a tube, Nancy's parents requested that doctors stop providing the nutrition that was sustaining her body. They based their request on what they believed Nancy would want if she were able to verbalize it. The parents' request advanced to the Missouri Supreme Court and was denied. In the court's opinion, no one could exercise Nancy's right to refuse treatment without "clear and convincing evidence." Eventually, the parents' request to stop artificial nutrition was granted by the state's probate court. Nancy Cruzan's life in a vegetative state began when she was 25. She died at age 33.

The Cruzan case helped to implement laws and create legal vehicles to respect and ensure a person's right to refuse treatment, even when stopping such treatment could lead to their death. In 1990 the Patient's Self-Determination Act (Levin, 1990) was passed into federal law. It required medical facilities that receive federal funds to protect a person's right to determine their healthcare decisions and honor their documented wishes.

The development of *My Voice – My Choice*

Gail, together with Chris Westphal, Father Leliaert, ethics committee member Kay Felt, JD, and others, took on the formidable task of developing the MVMC advance directive packet for the Oakwood system. Gail recalls the how MVMC took shape:

> Developing our own document really came about from our experiences meeting with families who had never communicated about end-of-life care or done the "what

---

3   *For more information on this case, see the Resources section at the end of the book.*

ifs." They had no clue where to go with the bad news they were getting. They told us they wished that they had had a conversation sooner before the bad news came. That was one of the first questions we would always ask those put in the position of making decisions for their loved one: "Did you talk about end of life before? Did your mom ever express any specific wishes?"

Sometimes information was gathered by remembering past conversations, like if their mom had said she never wanted to be in a nursing home. That told you something and gave us as staff a place to start a conversation. We could then reframe questions, and they would tell us more, such as, "She said it's important that she would be able to feed herself."

We decided it was important to include questions as part of our advance directive packet. They are so important because it really makes people think about specific circumstances, like how they would feel about not being able to feed themselves. It helped to bring out in the open what would or wouldn't be acceptable to them.

The discussion and documentation also helped relieve the spokesperson from having to guess. What a horrible thing to ask the families: "Well, if you don't know, can you guess?" In the event these conversations never took place, we would ask if they might surmise what their loved one would want based on their knowledge of how they led their life: "What was important to your mom? What did she believe in? Did she have religious or spiritual beliefs?"

All those things go hand in hand. Our staff's goal was to help them discover a loved one's personal wishes as well as give them the medical information to help them in making informed decisions.

The phrase *My Voice – My Choice* came from my life partner, Tom. He would hear me talk a lot about the question of futile continuation of care that would come to the ethics team. I called them the ugly end-of-life scenarios versus what I call a good end-of-life scenario. Tom would say, "Boy, you better use your voice before you lose your choice." That is how it started. Tom came up with the title.

Initial funding for MVMC came from the Masco Corporation's donation of $10,000. MVMC was also supported by Oakwood's Women's Volunteer Guild, the American Association of Critical Care Nurses, the Blue Cross Blue Shield of Michigan Foundation, and private contributors.

Another notable source of funding came from someone with a personal connection to this issue. When Gail was working at Oakwood as the head nurse in the CCU, she helped take care of Sally, a patient with multiple sclerosis who was wheelchair-bound and had severe heart issues. Sally intentionally overdosed because of the devastating progression of her disease. However, the overdose did not cause her death, but instead resulted in severe brain damage from anoxia.

The CCU protocol at that time was that life support must be continued if it was essential to keep someone alive. However, Sally had put in place a document that designated her husband as her power of attorney. The document also made clear that Sally did not want any aggressive treatment and did not want to be on a ventilator. The physician honored her wishes and life support was withdrawn. Gail remarked, "The doctor respected the law and clearly, that was a good thing."

Subsequently, Sally's husband gave Oakwood Hospital Foundation a significant financial donation that became a fund named in her memory. He wanted her fund to be used to promote conversation and documentation to ensure that a person's wishes regarding their medical care were honored. For many years the fund provided the means to reproduce *My Voice – My Choice*, which received the Michigan's Governor's Award of Excellence in 2002.

Essential components of an advance directive

There are three essential components of an advance directive for healthcare: the designation of the patient advocate, the designation of the treatment choices, and the patient advocate conversation.

Designating the patient advocate

Many advance directives that are available today include literature about how to choose an advocate (and backup advocate), as well as certain criteria that the advocate must meet. For example, the advocate must be 18 years or older, but does not have to be a relative. Advocates do not have to live in the same state, but must be reachable. Most notably, the advocate must sign a statement verifying that they will follow the patient's designated wishes. For this reason, it is important that the advocate is a person who can be trusted to follow documented decisions.

Often people believe there is an obligation to choose one's spouse as the advocate, but many people do not want to put their spouse in that position—not because the partner might "pull the plug" too soon, but rather that they wouldn't be able to withdraw treatment for any reason.

Gail knew her partner Tom would not be able to follow her very specific wishes. Her own advance directive makes it clear that under no circumstance should life-prolonging treatment be used. She does not want cardiac resuscitation or to be put on a ventilator. One of her daughters told Gail she would not be able to honor that request. Her other daughter agreed to become her advocate, although there needed to be many conversations to help her understand why this decision was important to her mother.

Joanne Lax, JD, who participated in many ethics consultations, emphasizes the importance of trust in choosing an advocate, saying, "Just find that person who you trust who is going to look at everything, know what your values are and try and follow them, and understand them in the nuanced situations that they need to be applied."

Dr. Reitemeier stresses how important it is for the person who is completing an advance directive to do as much as they can to explain to their advocate the "why" of their choices. Understanding why helps the advocate when unexpected circumstances may arise. In addition, he recommends that the document be routinely reviewed with the chosen advocate to account for changes in health or medical status. He explains:

> What you really have to do with an advance directive is to pick a surrogate decision- maker. That is the key. Inform them as best you can but then engage in what is called "adaptive decision-making." That is, "Given these new facts, given these new complications, this is now what I have decided. I know what I said I was going to decide before, but you know what, this is now a better informed, a more richly understood set of responses."

Designating the treatment choices

Advance directive documents provide an opportunity for a person to designate their preferred option of medical care/interventions if they are incapacitated with a critical illness. The person's choices can range from doing everything possible to preserve life, to refusing any life-sustaining treatment under any circumstances.

When considering an advance directive, people can be reluctant to lock themselves into a specific decision made in the present that they might feel differently about in the future. It is one of the main reasons people do not complete an advance directive.

Joanne Lax advises that the remedy for this is to gather as much information as possible:

> I think you want to talk to someone who can give you information about, well, if you say you don't want a ventilator, what is that really going to mean? What is kidney dialysis all about? What are the situations in which you would use it? Gather information to make sure you are informed and don't just make these meager statements because you think it's the thing to say, "I want no heroic measures." Make sure you know what you are talking about.

> One lesson learned is not to be too circumscribing in any document that you write. Try and make sure that there's enough opportunity for your decision-maker to assess the real "here and now" of your situation—socially, economically, medically, everything—before deciding. I think that's important.

Dr. Reitemeier explains how the mindset of many people who are trying to determine what sort of treatments they want can make the process of creating an advance directive more challenging:

> You walk into this advance directive writing as if you've got a rational linear set of preferences that are not going to be affected by the circumstances, or the context in which you learn about the circumstances. And in fact, it is just the opposite. You don't walk in with a preset of prioritized values; you walk in with a cluster, a cloudy cluster of values. And they get sorted out in response to the circumstances themselves.

Clarifying the "cloudy cluster of values" is an important precursor to making the choices that an advance directive documents. Communicating those values to the chosen advocate and explaining how they inform the choices documented in the advance directive helps the advocate and the healthcare provider apply them in future medical scenarios.

The patient advocate conversation: Communicating end-of-life wishes through values-based dialogue

Gail and the team of authors for MVMC recognized that talking about end-of-life wishes can be very difficult, both for the person completing the document as well as for their family members, who may be hesitant to ask their loved ones what their wishes might be. For that reason, they designed the MVMC advance directive not only as a legal document that captured a person's choices, but also as a comprehensive packet of information that provided educational material and prompts for in-depth discussion.

The packet contained a series of specific questions that asked the respondent to think about what they may or may not want in terms of medical treatments. It also encouraged dialogue with the patient advocate about why they made those choices. Incorporating the advocate's participation into the process of creating the advance directive helped better inform and prepare them for any decisions they may need to make in the future on the patient's behalf.

These questions the advance directive packet contained were inspired by the experiences that Gail and the team had as they helped patients close the circle. They were divided into categories representing different facets of the end-of-life experience. Here are some examples of the categories and questions used as prompts for discussion:

> **Physical Independence:** Is it important to me to be able to feed, bathe and toilet myself without depending on others?

> **Decision-Making:** Is it important to me to be told the truth about my condition and chances for recovery no matter how "bad" the news?

Social: Is it important to me to be able to talk with and understand others?

Aggressiveness of Treatment: Is it important for me to be allowed to die comfortably and free of machines if there is little hope of recovery?

The values-based conversation that these questions encouraged accomplished more than simply approving or rejecting specific treatments. Gail, FMSS staff, social workers, and chaplains who helped patients complete the form found that the questions led to deeper, more meaningful conversations between loved ones that identified not only when a continuation of life would no longer be acceptable, or to what lengths treatment should continue, but also why. The conversation would often segue into other significant topics, including relationships, which then prompted a deeper understanding between the participants. Martha witnessed the productive effects of MVMC both through Family Matters and as a teacher:

> One of the requirements for the Bachelor of Science in Nursing medical ethics class that I taught was to have each student assist a loved one complete an advance directive. The students were provided with the MVMC packet and were required to go through all the literature and to journal how the assignment went. In almost every case the students first expressed how difficult it was to introduce the topic but how the conversations that followed, aided by the prompts, were meaningful and in some cases enhanced relationships. For me, it is an indicator that these difficult discussions become an important step in eventually being able to help close the circle for someone you love.

Dr. Weber and his wife personally served as the patient advocates for their friend. Their experience demonstrates that the patient advocate conversation should be ongoing. He shared a challenge that they encountered:

> We know what she wants generally. We worked through the form with her. In fact, she did a couple of versions, because she is very focused on details. But ever since she did it, she has waffled when it comes to real issues, and she has accepted treatment that she previously said she didn't want. Even if she changes her mind, even if she doesn't always adhere to what she says she was going to adhere to, it's her right to change her mind.
>
> She wants to talk to us, but I think she wants us to be present as she talks it out and support her. So, it's her call, not ours. We can support her, we can support her by asking questions like, "Do you feel good about that, or do you have second thoughts?" Whatever sort of questions would help her process how much she is really thinking about the decision she is tending toward.
>
> So that's in the process of making up your mind. Even when you have an advance directive, I find…people don't always necessarily do what they say they are going to do.
>
> People change their mind when they are actually faced with it. They can say in advance that they don't want it. Just like I'm saying in advance I don't want such and such. But when you get there it's hard to let go. And that might be true…but you can't assume that.

As Dr. Weber discovered, even after MVMC or another advance medical directive has been completed, it's important for advocates to continue to check in with their friend or family member to make sure that they still understand the person's wishes and will be able to uphold them if called upon to do so.

Advance directive document review: A physician's ethical responsibility

The Patient Self-Determination Act requires healthcare facilities to inquire if a patient has created an advance directive and to educate patients about them. In addition, a provision of Medicare/Medicaid funding requires that hospitals address advance directives with patients, add them to the medical record, and implement them in the plan of care when necessary. Whether you are an admitting physician, bedside nurse, or a social worker in a case management department, it is essential to review a patient's advance directive and be aware of the components that must be present to make it a legal document. Some healthcare systems even have a required process in the electronic medical record to document that the advance directive was reviewed.

Gail and her team developed several procedures to assist the Oakwood system in meeting the federal and Medicare/Medicaid requirements for advance directives:

- Staff asked a patient on admission if they had an advance directive and documented the response.

- If the patient had an advance directive, FMSS staff reviewed it to make sure it met the legal requirements and confirmed the patient's wishes as currently correct.

- FMSS ensured the physicians and healthcare team were aware of the advance directive.

- If the patient did not have an advance directive, FMSS provided education about the advance directive and would help the patient complete it if possible.

Shifting circumstances can result in a patient changing their choices. If the patient indicated that there should be a change of advocate or treatment choice, FMSS helped them create a new, accurate advance directive.

It cannot be stressed enough that attending physicians have an enormous fiduciary (ethical) responsibility to be aware of the wishes of the patient and to honor them to the best of their ability, while still following set standards of medically appropriate care. In the event that a treatment does not provide a medical benefit for a patient or merely prolongs an existence the patient had indicated would be unacceptable, it is the professional responsibility of the physician to inform the advocate that continued treatment no longer aligns with the patient's wishes.

Patient or patient advocate: Who decides?

If a patient is confused, critically ill, or otherwise impaired the medical team has the task of determining if the patient can make their own medical decisions. In these cases, a neurologist, psychiatrist, or gerontologist will be consulted to assess a patient's capacity for medical decision-making. Unless these experts determine that the patient is medically incapable of making decisions for themselves, the patient is always approached as the primary decision-maker.

It is important that the patient advocate understands that their role as the decision-maker takes place only when the patient is no longer capable of expressing their own wishes. Martha has observed advocates who were unclear on this point:

> The daughter of a patient approached me in the hallway. She was crying and stressed because her mother's condition was deteriorating, and she was trying to decide if further aggressive treatment should be continued. The daughter, who was the advocate, had the advance directive document in her hand. What decision should she make based on the document?

But I asked if her mother was still capable of understanding what was going on, and her response was yes. So, we went in together to talk to her mother and see if she understood the situation and ask what treatment she would or would not want. It's important to remember that a patient's real-time choices always take precedence over what is documented in the [advance directive]. Treatment choice is first and foremost their own decision. The daughter was relieved to have support for both her mother and herself and a better understanding of navigating her own role in what could be a life-altering decision.

If a patient's mental competency is compromised or serious illness prohibits their ability to make medical decisions, the advance directive comes into play and the named advocate steps into the role of decision-maker. One of the greatest benefits of completing an advance directive document is that it ensures that the patient has specifically chosen the person who will be making decisions on their behalf, and that person is then obligated to follow their wishes. The document also clarifies the patient's choices for the advocate and unburdens the family of determining who is responsible for decisions.

But sometimes even with an advance directive, issues can arise. For instance, designated advocates can themselves become ill or mentally compromised, or pass away. If any of these things happen, a successor or back-up advocate must step in. Beyond being medically unable to serve as patient advocate, some advocates encounter other barriers. Gail encountered situations in which a chosen advocate confessed they could not follow the wishes they once agreed to follow and refused to participate as the patient's decision-maker. In those cases, if a successor advocate has not been named, the staff would often seek a consensus from the family. Many scenarios are possible, which underscores how important it is for medical staff to review the document and to give themselves time to sort out any possible issue that could present itself.

It was often a tremendous personal relief for the advocate to recognize that their duty to the patient was to follow the patient's wishes, even if it meant the withdrawal of care. In fact, when Gail went to the bedside, or out into the community to educate and encourage others to complete advance directives, she would always tell people, "This is the best gift you can give your family. It takes away the burden they feel of not knowing what you want. It relieves them of the guilt of guessing."

Gail recalls a particular case with a remarkable outcome that powerfully demonstrated the positive impact an advance directive can have, both on a patient and on the patient's relationships:

> I helped a patient I will call "Bill." He was probably in his early 30s and mentally challenged. At least that is what was put on the chart. Did that mean he can make decisions or he can't make decisions? It can be a fine line when one doctor assesses his capacity one way, and a few others are saying, "Well no, he kind of gets it."
>
> Ethics was called in. Bill had four sisters who were lawyers. He had been trying to make decisions about his end of life but they were trying to speak for him. When I got to the room they were all there.
>
> Bill was a charming guy. He was sitting in the hospital chair and we shook hands and I just sat down and started to talk to him in generalities so I could get to know him. Quite frankly I found him to be really sharp. He appeared to comprehend and process everything we talked about. When I told him I understood he wanted to do an advance directive, he said, "Absolutely." I brought out the MVMC packet and told him I would go through every page with him and if he had any questions I would answer them right then and there. It took us over two hours.

There wasn't a peep in that room from his sisters. They were in awe of not only the document but about Bill talking about his choices. I think he felt free to talk and this was his chance. He felt empowered to make his own choices. The more I got into the discussion with him the more I believed that he was confident and competent.

Because I believed in autonomy and the right to make one's own choices, I went into the room with an open mind. Was Bill able to understand the consequences if he chose not to have something done? He said he did not want to be intubated. He had been intubated before and didn't want any part of that happening again. He told me, "I've been there and I don't want it anymore." It made sense to me and it was powerful. The tears started streaming down from his sisters' faces. There was a brand new, fresh relationship that was given birth in that room and I will never forget it.

We completed the document together. It took a long time. He felt good about it and started crying and wanted to hug and thank me. I think that was one of the first meaningful and full conversations he'd been able to have with his family about certain choices. I made sure to do a lot of "what if" questions with him. He had very concrete opinions and to me they were logical and made sense.

When I asked him who he wanted to be his advocate and successor advocate he gave me four reasons why they were his choice. He went above and beyond what most people would have reasoned. His sisters were all quite impressed. They were appreciative that I had wanted them there to witness the process. I told them they were part of it and Bill wanted them to be part of it and that they needed to hear what he had to say. This was one of the advance directive sessions that I cherish the most in my career. It was one of the most spiritual moments.

A patient advocate's promise

Sometimes when a legal document is done in an attorney's office as part of a last will and testament, it names an advocate but does not include a discussion with the advocate about the person's end-of-life wishes. This can be traumatizing to the advocate if they are faced with medical decision-making. Gail's team experienced several cases in which the legal advocate had no idea they were even named as a decision-maker.

One Family Matters case that led to an ethics consult highlights how profoundly important an advance directive is for an unresponsive patient in the critical care unit. "Jane" was an elderly patient who had a major stroke that left her in a vegetative state and on full life support. She was a single person who had been a librarian for many years and did not have any relatives. Her only recorded contacts were her two friends, one of whom had passed away. Hospital staff contacted Jane's remaining friend, but she was also elderly and said it would be too difficult to visit. Family Matters staff called and updated her daily.

The ethics committee was consulted to give its recommendation on next steps, as Jane was heading toward a tracheostomy and PEG tube and a long-term care facility. Ethics committee member Joanne Lax's connection with the legal community was of tremendous value in this case:

> There had been talk there might be an advance directive, but nobody could find it. As it turned out we did a bunch of sleuthing and then the friend informed us that the patient had a lawyer, and the lawyer had the advance directive. I was able to contact the lawyer and he provided us with her documentation. The person who was named as the advocate in the advance directive was this same friend we had been speaking with, but because it had been done so long ago, she had forgotten she was the advocate.

In previous phone conversations with staff, she said she didn't want to get involved and she wasn't going to help make any decisions.

The recovered document clearly stated that Jane would not want to be kept alive by artificial means and it gave the legal authority of her advocate to stop treatment. Although it was difficult for the friend to step into the role of advocate, she finally agreed to fulfill the promise she made to the patient many years before. Jane's wishes were followed because they were clearly documented, because the advocate was ultimately willing to step in as the decision-maker, and because of the extra effort made by the ethics team to find the directive and support the advocate in her role.

The FMSS team observed many similar situations in which an advocate, understanding their responsibility and promise, fulfilled their role and followed a patient's directive. Knowing and then following a patient's own personal choices can help to alleviate uncertainty and help temper the sadness and grief that occurs when a patient dies. An advance directive can also help prevent a fracture in the family over conflicting opinions on treatment or indecision regarding what to do.

In the absence of an advance directive

There are many cases in which there is no advance directive document and family is called on to make choices on the patient's behalf. If the patient offered no prior guidance about their end-of-life wishes, then a reflection on past experiences and conversations with the patient, or knowledge of their personal, religious, and cultural beliefs can be used to help support decision-making. This sort of evaluation that encourages making choices based on what is known about the patient and what they might choose is called the *substituted judgment standard* (Jaworska, 2009). The *best interests standard* is another criteria used for decision-making and utilized if there is no information about a patient's preferences. This standard takes into consideration what "most people" would want for themselves under the given circumstances, based on harms or benefits, and any decisions for the patient are made accordingly.

While these alternatives exist, they are less effective than an advance directive like *My Voice - My Choice*. The Covid pandemic of 2019-2020 is a good example of the need for an advance directive. In 2019, especially before the vaccine was available, patients were being admitted into critical care units and quickly declining. The medical staff needed to be clear of who was the patient's choice of surrogate decision maker and asked patients upon admission to designate someone. A conversation about their wishes was not always possible due to the emergent nature of the admission or sudden decline that led to intubation. In these cases, the staff counted on the family member to make a decision based on a substitute judgement or best interest standard.

Another strong argument for an advance directive is that it reflects the patient's own express wishes for their medical care. This prevents the possibility of a family member making a treatment decision based on their own self-interest rather than the best interest of a patient. A heartbreaking example of this was "Charlie," the diabetic patient who was suffering from severe sepsis and had had multiple amputations. Despite his poor prognosis and the gangrene spreading throughout his body, his wife insisted upon continuing treatment. This case highlights how other people's self-interest can impact a patient's end-of-life care. If Charlie was able to speak for himself, or had an advance directive, it could have prevented what Gail would call an ugly death.

Gail strongly advocates that everyone complete an advance directive because she saw the positive difference it made for patients and their families in closing the circle. But she also acknowledges that completing an advance directive is not easy:

There are a myriad of issues around end-of-life that are so personal. I think there are great fears around it and people change their mind about what they might want. I think there are fears even when you have made decisions, like I have, about not wanting a lot of aggressive therapies at the end of life. You can change your mind and everybody has to keep an open mind…It's ok.

It makes it a lot harder when you try to communicate with family what your wishes are, and they don't agree with them. That brings forth a whole new uncontrolled anxiety because then you wonder if you have the wrong advocate. Do I need to go to someone else that will agree and will follow my wishes? It is a very complex thing and I think, as we get older it may be harder because we are closer to death…

Trying to help people have that conversation is a hard thing to do for a lot of families, for most of us. Even the ones who have been out there and done it, it's still hard when it comes right down to that time and it's your family and your life and your end-of-life journey.

Despite these challenges, Gail believes that having an advance directive document often determined the quality of the patient's death:

Over time, as I witnessed what I call the good, bad and ugly death, I started thinking, what made this death a good death? Why did I say it was a good death? Nine out of ten times it's because the family had had a conversation and even more, some of them had some legal documents that provided us with the spokesperson who was supposed to know what the wishes were.

Wow, what a beautiful journey that was. No fighting, no guessing, no wondering, no sitting around the table trying to yank information out of a family that is trying to grieve and you are just trying to find out the wishes of their loved one. That could be awful. So, I think what occurred to me at that time [was] that this kind of communication, along with documentation of some sort, was needed. Everybody needs one and how can we do that? …

It was just the beginning of years and years of work on the advance directive: *My Voice – My Choice.* I think that is where it all started, and with good reason.

Join our Circle

- Gail believes strongly that everyone should capture their end-of-life wishes in a formal legal document and select a patient advocate that can be trusted to see that those wishes are followed. **Have you told anyone what your wishes would be for end-of-life care? Do you have an advance directive? If so, how did it feel to go through that process? If you don't have one yet, what might be holding you back?**

- Gail and her team developed several procedures to assist the Oakwood system in meeting the federal and Medicare/Medicaid requirements for advance directives. **What procedures are in place at your hospital to determine if a patient has an advance directive? How is the healthcare team made aware of the patient's advance directive and the end-of-life wishes it contains? What role do you play to promote this process?**

- When considering an advance directive, people can be reluctant to lock themselves into a specific decision made in the present that they might feel differently about in the future. Joanne Lax advises that the remedy for this is to gather as much information as possible. **What other ways could you address this concern with patients who are reluctant to create an advance directive?**

- The MVMC advance directive packet contains a series of questions representing different facets of the end-of-life experience. These questions are meant to prompt a values-based conversation between patient and patient advocate about the "why" behind the patient's treatment choices. **Have you talked to your loved one/parents/family about what sort of treatments they may or may not want? Have you discussed the reasons behind their decisions?**

Spiritual Support, Palliative Care and Hospice Care: Paths Toward Comfort and Meaning

You matter because you are you, and you matter to the end of your life. We will do all we can not only to help you die peacefully, but also to live until you die.

—Cicely Saunders, founder of hospice and palliative care

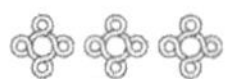

Everyone's journey toward closing the circle is unique. As healthcare providers, we adapt our approach to each patient to honor their needs and assist their transition physically and emotionally. It is likely that your hospital, like Oakwood, has a range of resources that you can offer to assist patients at end of life. Advance medical directives like My Voice - My Choice *are among the most important resources available because they allow patients to document their treatment preferences. In addition to advance directives, healthcare providers at Oakwood also offered patients spiritual support, palliative care, and hospice care.*

As we discuss the value of each of these options, we include our own personal experiences with them. Gail, Martha, Ann, and many of those in the Family Matters community have supported their loved ones' end-of-life journeys. Our firsthand accounts offer insight into end-of-life care not only as healthcare providers but as spouses, parents, children, and friends. We hope that our stories illustrate the value of these three resources and show how they can help your patients "live until they die."

When a patient's curative options are limited or have been

exhausted, there are three disciplines that have a lot to offer those approaching end of life: spiritual support, palliative care, and hospice. Not all hospitals have a spiritual support department, but for those that do, its services can be requested by patients and families at any time during admission. However, it is most often called upon during a healthcare crisis or at the end of life. Palliative care is an interdisciplinary specialty that can assist patients with poor prognosis, life-limiting diseases, and end-stage chronic illnesses such as COPD and CHF. A palliative care provider's goal is to manage symptoms and provide treatments that will optimize a patient's wellbeing for as long as it is feasible. Hospice care is also interdisciplinary and focuses on comfort measures for those who have an end-stage terminal illness with a prognosis of six months or less.

Although our attention is primarily on patients in the critical care units, the professionals in these fields use their expertise to provide resources and comfort care options throughout the inpatient setting.

The value of spiritual support

The concept of spirituality is found in all cultures and societies. It is expressed in an individual's search for ultimate meaning through participation in religion and/or belief in God, family, naturalism, humanism, and the arts. All these factors can influence how patients and health care professionals perceive health and illness and how they interact with one another. (Puchalski et al, 1999, p. 25)

Spiritual support departments serve the entire hospital population: the patients, families, and staff. It is a common misconception that chaplains only meet with religious patients or offer specific religious teachings. Rather, chaplains respect diverse religious practices. Their fundamental role is to provide support for patients' spiritual needs.

Rev. Marshall explains his approach to meeting a person's spiritual needs:

> It is that transition from religion to spirituality. I am a firm believer that everybody is spiritual. Whether you like kittens or puppies, you are a spiritual person. You see value and beauty in something. I want to tap into that when I work with patients. That is where we connect. That is what drew me into this field. That is what kept me but that is also what was very challenging.
>
> One of the things that makes chaplaincy difficult is that probably 70%, maybe even 80% of what we do is with end of life. Everyone who comes into the hospital has the moment when they think, *Am I going home? Is this going to go bad?* But when things tend to go well, they say, "Nice to see you, Chaplain…and let us move on." It is when things have the possibility of going bad that people really want to talk to a chaplain. They want to air this stuff out. They want to get things out. That is when we become involved.
>
> So, I think it is very important that we meet people where they are and find out, knowing where they are, what is important to them, and what means the most to them. Where is their purpose, their meaning, and their value? Then, we address those things and how we can enhance them with the time that we have. When you do it that way, you will see that everybody is different.
>
> I did some hospice work with a guy who just wanted to turn his motorcycle on. So that is what we did. I am not a motorcycle guy, but I learned how to crank it up. We cranked it up and we let it rev and that made his day. He would be fine until I came to see him again because that was his spirituality. Singing a hymn would not do anything for him, but that vroom did everything for him.
>
> We all have meaning. Something matters to us. And I

think as ministers and clinicians we need to see what matters and how we can connect and enhance that.

If finding meaning is the essence of spirituality, then whether it is expressed in traditional or non-traditional avenues, a chaplain's ability to acknowledge and honor that meaning can help a patient close the circle and achieve a good death.

Father Richard Leliaert would agree that being a good chaplain is not about promoting a particular religion. During Father Leliaert's work in hospitals, some people saw his white collar and immediately told him that they did not have a religious practice:

> When I would come into the room, I would say, "I am here to talk with you and meet you because you are the kind of person that is interesting to talk to. Let us talk together."

> There was one man I especially remember who did not believe in God, but he did not put me off. He really talked about living and dying. Instead of trying to get a person to believe in God or to repent of sins, or talk about heaven, we just talked about, "Tell me, what is meaningful to you in your life? How would you say to people that you have had a meaningful life?"

According to Father Leliaert, good chaplains are good listeners. In the classroom, he taught his students that there is a reason we have two ears and only one mouth. Father Leliaert's experience with chaplaincy also taught him the importance of humility and the true nature of wisdom:

> It is about basic humility in facing the issues of life and death. We do not handle them or manhandle them; there is a dynamic here that transcends our ability to control it or to force it.

> I think other than humility, my perspective of death and dying has a lot to do with wisdom and the difference

between knowing and being wise. They are related, but they are very distinct. If somebody were to ask, "What is the difference?": I treasure knowledge. But no matter how much I know, it does not automatically make me wise. So, death and dying was a real course that is always lifelong, and there are a lot of credits, mainly your whole life. But a certain amount of wisdom will guide you every day in ways that keep you open to what really matters, and the wisdom to know what really matters.

In Father Richard's experience, the need for closure at the end of life can take unexpected turns. He gives as an example the husband who learned, as his wife was dying, that his beloved daughter was not biologically his:

> You see a lot at the end of life. It is not so much just getting them ready for death but [for them] to seek healing and forgiveness so there's peace between family members, peace between God and the dying person.

Gail witnessed how the support and attentiveness offered by Father Richard and other chaplains assisted both patients and staff regardless of their religious affiliations:

> When I think about how many times, no matter what their faith was, if I were doing CPR on a patient, I would ask my nurses to page Father Rich. If he were not there, Phyllis Miller, who also was a chaplain, would have come.
>
> I do not know if Father Rich knew how much he really helped. He helped me and helped the families. Trying to resuscitate someone is such a critical moment and a tense moment and he helped a lot of people. It did not matter what religion they were; he was calming and gave them excellent support. He is really a smart man. I love Father Rich. I could not count how many times he sat in on meetings with myself and the doctors. He would just sit there quietly listening to all sides of the issue and he

would barely chime in until I would ask him, "Father Rich, what do you think?" He always had words of support and comfort. He is a beautiful man.

Although Gail does not follow an organized religion, many healthcare providers of varying religious beliefs and backgrounds lean on their own spirituality to support their work with end-of-life patients. Dr. Hnatiuk carried a printed card, "A Physician's Prayer," in his wallet for the entirety of his practice and up to the time of his own death in 2023. It was well worn with use, as he recited it daily:

> Do I pray for patients? Yes, I pray in general. I include them in my prayers because I'm a Catholic and I say prayers in the evening, and I go to Mass. So, I pray for everybody. I visit the sick. It's part of the things you do.
>
> Do I pray for specific patients? There have been a few that I have prayed for. I pray that they either miraculously recover or sometimes I pray that they would die and no longer suffer.

Mary Catherine Wright, RN, is also a practicing Christian. She is extremely comfortable in her spiritual skin, and she believes that spirituality and end-of-life care are inextricable:

> Spirituality? That is the only way you can do it. People say, "Oh, you do hospice or Family Matters? How do you do it? Doesn't it wear you out?" I would say that sometimes it did. But really, I always felt when I was meeting with the family and the tide turned [toward hospice and comfort measures], in a way we thought was best for the patient, that it was really a spiritual moment and that I was privileged to be there with them. The Lord Jesus was right there with us, you know, where two or more are gathered, He is there. So, it's very spiritual, very spiritual.

Chris Westphal relates there were several cases in which the medically unexplainable occurred during her years of practice. She categorizes these events as spiritually significant:

> I had this one case when the lady was elderly, minimally responsive, and the family was gathering. We talked about how they might make the most of the time. And then the grandson came, and he was playing country western music. She sat up, and she put her arms around him, and they "danced" while she sat up in bed. That night, she died. The family told everyone, "You would not believe what happened!"

> There are miracles that happen. It may not be a recovery per se but there are things that happen that are beyond comprehension.

When asked about the role of spirituality in his practice, Dr. Haydon reveals that he has begun to introduce the topic more often and to embrace the concept of spirituality in his work with patients and family:

> I find I am bringing spirituality up a little bit more. I do acknowledge the fact that I need to be humble. I do not know it all. I hope I have been given the tools, and I have been blessed in that regard, and that we are all working together, and that God might be part of that team. I would like to open it up, so it is OK to talk about. And I find I am doing that more. I do not know why.

Addressing spirituality at the end of life is not in every healthcare provider's comfort zone. Dr. Bair identifies as an atheist. However, he recognizes the importance of spiritual support in his neonatal unit, not only for the parents of the babies, but also for the nursing staff who care for and bond with these tiny and fragile infants.

While healthcare providers take different approaches toward spirituality in their own lives and work with patients of diverse religious beliefs, spirituality is often an integral part of end-of-life care. Martha Hnatiuk, who is at ease with spirituality and its many faces, at first had difficulty approaching patients or family members to ask if they would like someone from spiritual support to come and visit them. She believes that her initial hesitancy was based on fear that people would think she would be judgmental if they declined, that her question could be viewed as an intrusion on their privacy, or that they would be alarmed by the proposition.

But with time she recognized that it was best to directly ask the patient or family if they would like to see someone from spiritual support because she knew this service could bring closure, or relieve stress, or provide guidance. It was not a question that should be neglected or avoided—there were profound benefits the department offered. The chaplains and volunteers in the Spiritual Support Department covered all areas of the hospital, made rounds daily, and were available day and night for interventions requested by family, staff, and patients. They were often present at family meetings. There were countless instances when the hospital chaplains or the department's volunteer staff offered compassionate emotional and spiritual care either during a crisis or in the final hours of a patient's life.

Families were also encouraged to invite their own faith leader to attend critical decision-making meetings. This was particularly important for Catholic, Muslim, and Jehovah's Witnesses patients whose family members wanted guidance from their own faith leader concerning what treatments were acceptable in their specific religious teachings.

Although spiritual support is not the primary focus of either palliative care or hospice care, both include a spiritual support professional as one of their team members.

Palliative care

Palliative care is a specialized service to manage symptom control and enhance a person's quality of life when an illness becomes serious, chronic, or life-threatening. It helps patients dealing with nausea, pain, or whatever problematic symptoms may arise. Palliative care also provides support for the patient's family and assists with healthcare decision-making.

Many primary care physicians practice palliative care themselves by addressing symptoms, prescribing medications, and providing treatments as a disease progresses. However, when finding a cure is no longer possible and the medical goal is primarily symptom control or providing treatments that may help alleviate problems, the attending physician may choose to utilize a palliative care service. This service is designed specifically for the intermediary stage between chronic health problems and the inevitable decline of the patient, with the goal of helping patients optimize their quality of life. Dr. Mohs explains this transition:

> Most of the time the primary care physicians are successful in normal situations with families and patients. But there are times when it gets really complicated and really rough. There are times when the physician, frankly, doesn't have as much time as the situation calls for to really be able to communicate what the healthcare team needs to communicate in terms of prognosis and treatment options. They don't necessarily have the time to listen to what the family is going through, what the patient is going through, what this means for their life, and how we can match up what we have to offer from healthcare to help dampen an often tragic impact of a disease process. So palliative care can be that added benefit when it gets more complicated or when, for example, a symptom needs more focused attention.

Depending on the resources and needs of a hospital, there may be a single palliative care practitioner, or a team of professionals. When Dr. Mohs was the palliative care physician for Oakwood, her original team consisted of herself and a nurse practitioner. She enthusiastically reported on how the service grew: "Now we have a chaplain, a social worker and three full-time and one half-time nurse practitioners. It is a full team."

Chris Westphal was the first palliative care nurse practitioner who worked alongside Dr. Mohs. She often took on the task of describing palliative care to patients at their first meeting. She explained it to them as a combination of three dimensions of care:

> Our goal is to help you to live as well as possible with your illness by doing three things. [The first is] making sure we understand how you want to live [and] what is important to you, and working together so that our care is consistent with that. The next is to make sure that we can address those symptoms, whether it's your physical symptoms, emotional struggles, or family needs. And the third is figuring out the resources. Those are the three things: goals, symptoms, and resources. We are here in the hospital, and we can tap into resources here, but you will leave, and you will go back home. So, what can we put in place to help you when you go back home?

Palliative care can follow a patient for years, with an interdisciplinary team helping the family and patient navigate illness until the ongoing treatment becomes burdensome or ineffectual and it is time to pivot to comfort care, or hospice.

Dr. Mohs explains the difference between palliative care and hospice care and when the transition should take place:

> Palliative care can be really early on in any health issue trajectory. It can be really early on in a disease process that's temporary and the person is going to live a normal life span. It can also be really early on in something that

we know will end in the person's death in either two weeks or two years or five years, but we can see it as a terminal disease.

Let's say, small cell lung cancer. In the very beginning you are uncertain how this is going to go but the evidence suggests that if you get treatment and you can tolerate the treatment, if you are coming in with a good functional status, then you are going to get full remission status for at least a couple of years. That is what you are looking at. So palliative care can be there at the beginning to make sure symptoms are controlled during chemotherapy…

If the therapy doesn't go well and it turns out you are not going to make it through the chemotherapy, through the treatment, [the] palliative care service…can help the family start adjusting to that, the patient adjust to that, and take their cues and at the same time educate them and move them in the direction of hospice. Sometimes people never go to hospice. They die. I believe sometimes people think that if they don't go to hospice they won't die, which unfortunately isn't true.

Chris Westphal provides an excellent example of moving from palliative to hospice care with her own father's course of illness. She had years of experience working with hospice partners at Oakwood. Her father was the beneficiary of her knowledge when he was approaching the end of his life and looked to her for guidance. He was 92 and receiving palliative care while still going to the casino and socializing with his lady friend. But eventually he began making frequent trips to the hospital, followed by time spent in a rehab facility for physical and occupational therapy. She knew that this revolving door would continue without resolving his underlying health issues:

When my dad first came home, we talked about hospice.

He did PT/OT and used that benefit, and it optimized him. Finally, I thought we had optimized as far as we were going to go, and I kept worrying about him having a crisis and being readmitted to the hospital. He told me, "I do not want any more procedures. I do not want a pacemaker." The hospice nurse came to us and said, "All right, what is your goal?" He said, "I want to party every day."

Chris's father continued under hospice care to "party" in his assisted living facility, watching baseball and football, discussing current events, and hanging out with his girlfriend. He closed his circle on his own terms, with the support of hospice and those who loved him, pursuing what made life meaningful for him.

Hospice care

In general, a hospice patient is someone diagnosed with a life-limiting illness who has decided to forgo life-prolonging measures and focus on being kept comfortable for their remaining time. In critical care units, physicians or palliative care staff usually begin the conversation about the transition to hospice care. It may take several meetings to educate the patient and family about what services hospice offers. Sometimes, that discussion takes place when the discharge plan is being formulated by the medical team and patient and family. If the patient is transitioning to care at home, hospice is an option that provides important resources for both the patient and their family.

In the hospital, a hospice consultation is initiated by the medical team as a written order in the patient's chart. Patients and families can also request information at any time from social workers during their inpatient stay.

Many hospitals have designated social work staff to address hospice consults. In addition, they may have contracts with hospice providers to meet patients at their bedside. The social work staff will first meet with the patient and family to discuss their understanding of hospice and the choices of hospice providers in their geographic area. Ann Caulfield-Cook, whose PhD is in social work, describes the role of the social worker at the initial meeting:

> Social workers are often the first staff to discuss hospice care at length with a patient and/or family. They will assess how much the patient or family member knows about hospice care. Sometimes, patients misunderstand what hospice care is, believing hospice care means the withdrawal of all medical care. So, usually, the conversation starts with an explanation of the services offered by hospice.

Once the social worker has met with a patient and/or family member and they agree to a specific hospice provider, the hospice provider's intake nurse will contact the family. The hospice intake nurse will determine if the patient qualifies for hospice and where the care will be provided. Hospice care can take place at home or in extended care facilities. Home hospice is a valuable service for families that would never consider a nursing home for their loved one. Many families have cultural values that encourage caring for elderly loved ones in the home. There are hospice residential centers where the patient can stay until their death, but these facilities are limited in number. For example, there are only two in the Metro Detroit region where Oakwood Hospital is located.

A patient can also receive hospice care while in the hospital. This typically occurs when the hospice staff determines the patient is actively dying and needs comfort care measures, such as pain management, that would be best administered in the hospital setting. The hospice interdisciplinary team becomes the team guiding the patient's plan of care to help make the patient comfortable at the end of their life.

The value of hospice

Gail sees the value of hospice care when she compares the end-of-life experiences of her mother and her father:

> My mom had Parkinson's and always swore she never wanted to be in a nursing home. She would say, "Leave me alone, do not ever intubate me." We never did that, but she did end up in a nursing home because it was too much for my father to take care of her. She was delusional and hallucinating at home, and it was hard on my dad. I remember my partner Tom and I going over to the house. She was just so fragile, and Tom picked her up, and we had to take her to a nursing home. That is something that I swore I would never do. In reflection, if we both could have stopped working, I would have.

> My mom was not mentally there, and I had a really hard time looking at her. She was not my mom anymore. She got septic and was all contracted. Each day, I felt guilty. Thank God it was finally my dad who took charge and so I was just able to follow his lead. He loved my mom dearly, and they were a very strong couple. One day, he finally looked at the doctors and said, "That is it." We had gone too far as it is. She did not want any of this.

When Gail's father passed at the age of 93, he was under hospice care while he was living in the home she and Tom shared:

> It was exactly the opposite of my mom's case. He was so alert and so sharp and very grateful that we had taken him in. He started living with us when one day he had a fever, and I took him home for the night. He stayed with us for three years.

> They were wonderful, wonderful years. I felt like I was giving back to him all that he had given us as a family. To me, it was very, very meaningful to be able to give back. While living with us, he would sit in the TV chair, a big

leather rocking chair, and loved to read his stocks. I had aides in during the day because Tom and I both continued to work. One morning, we just found him in bed, and he passed. It was a stark difference from what we went through with my mom. His was a good death.

Dr. Bair similarly experienced the value that hospice care workers can provide at end of life. In his case, the hospice nurse provided care and relief not just for his mother, the patient, but also for himself and his brother as family members:

My brother and I were having this argument over and over: "Ok, if Mom is going to be like this"—and she was in a bad way, she could not respond, her eyes deviated, her face was all contorted, and she could not move—I was like, "Ok, are we talking feeding tube? Do we feed her, do we not feed her?" We talked about how she is already dehydrated and has kidney issues. And then hospice came in, and that took all the pressure off us. They were amazing.

They had [a nurse from hospice] come over, and they met with us, and they said, "Your mother is in the active phase of dying."

Here, I'm a doctor, and I had no idea what they were talking about. I said, "The active phase of dying? What do you mean?"

She said, "Well, your mother's dying."

I said, "Well, we're all dying." I was being smart-ass about it.

She said, "Your mother is going to be dead soon."

I asked, "How soon?"

She said, "There's nothing to be done, and your mother is going to be dead in the next four days."

They were off a bit. She died four hours later. She just suddenly stopped breathing.

Dr. Mohs, Chris Westphal, and Mary Catherine Wright all experienced how sensitive presenting hospice to patients and their families could be. While many people have had positive experiences with hospice care for their loved ones, there are mixed feelings about it. As Mary Catherine notes:

> Sometimes, it was hard to get the family to even talk about hospice; it was like the "H- word." I learned from Family Matters to give people time. In the beginning of working in hospice I thought we must tell patients they are in hospice [even] when family members would insist that we not tell them. But then, as I dug deeper with the family, I realized they wanted to tell them, but they just did not know how. In Family Matters, where I learned a lot about communication, I would be gentle and say, "I will be with you, or, if you want me to tell him, I will tell him."

Mary Catherine had two personal experiences that led to her wanting to help others talk honestly about hospice. As described in Chapter 5, when Mary Catherine was 19, she and her siblings suffered unnecessarily when no one communicated the reality of her mother's condition before she died. Another experience involved her beloved mother-in-law. After her mother-in-law fell ill, Mary Catherine believed she should be in hospice. She wanted to help her in-laws with the decision, but she was never invited to be a part of the conversation.

In contrast, as the advocate of her 94-year-old uncle, she was able to convey what hospice could provide for him, but without naming it:

> In my own family, my uncle was 94 years old, and he was dying. I had to fly out to Florida. It was my Uncle Kevin who was a mentor to me. With this situation I used all my

experience and what I had learned. I knew I did not have to ask him when they came to sign him on to hospice, "Is it ok if we sign you on to hospice?" He could not eat. He was throwing up. He could not eat for weeks. I did not want to hide it from him, but I did not want to put the burden on him. So, when the hospice nurse came, she gave him a brochure, and he read it. He never said to me, "It is ok. I want to sign up." But he read it. He was a librarian. He just put it down, and he was ok with it. That was all right with me. I did not hide it from him, but I did not have the need to say to him, "Uncle Kevin, is it ok if I sign you into hospice?" He trusted me.

Mary Catherine's professional experiences reflect how hospice care takes a special type of healthcare provider. As a hospice nurse, she rose to the challenges of a unique hospice situation, and helped a patient close the circle in a way that was profoundly meaningful to everyone involved.

During her work with a hospice provider, Mary Catherine was notified of a 60-year-old patient who was a drug addict. He had been homeless, but he was living in a hotel with a roommate who was on and off being clean. The hotel was in a bad neighborhood, so Mary Catherine initially met him and his roommate at the hospital:

> [I said] we would take him as a patient, but they both had to listen to me, or I was going to open up a can of whoop ass on them. [*Laughter*] He had to agree to work with us because we needed to get methadone. He was really tough. He was from the street, but he agreed. So, like I said before, you have to meet the person where they're at.

Mary Catherine was the only hospice worker who would agree to go to the patient's hotel. Other hospice nurses did not want to go there because there were bedbugs. The patient's situation caused additional challenges:

We had to have the narcotics in a lockbox because we did not want the patient taking it without supervision.

The roommate told me taking care of the patient was too much, and he couldn't handle it, and I said, "Whoa, you have to; he's got nobody else." We couldn't find any of the family. The social worker had given up and said she could not find any family.

Mary Catherine did everything she could to meet the patient's needs:

We got an employee that I worked with to get a friend she knew who was a hairdresser [to come] to the hotel. There were bedbugs, but since it was cold out, [the patient] could not go outside. But she cut his hair. He really didn't talk a lot about stuff, but he knew he was dying. She gave him a haircut and he had tears coming down his face. Because someone was kind enough to cut his hair.

As his hospice care continued, Mary Catherine's relationship with both the patient and his roommate grew. She brought in pizza for them, and would pick up things for them from the Salvation Army, like clean sheets:

I told the roommate that he had to help us keep things clean. One day, I went there, and there was blood on the pillowcase, and I was fussing about it, and the roommate said, "Man, I told you she was going to fuss at us about this dirty pillowcase! I told you!" [*Laughter*] So, I had to go back to the Salvation Army and get some more.

The patient died a peaceful death. Mary Catherine was able to locate his stepmom and sister, and organized a memorial service. Her experience with him had a profound effect both on her personally and on the organization she was part of:

That was a tough case. I ended up changing the culture at that hospice organization. I told them that we must go in and help. [If] he needs a bath, [we] are just going to have to gown up and go in and give that guy a bath. So, they did.

That was really all about communication, communication, and seeing [them] where they are at. It was a bad motel. People were looking at me, so I had my tough look on. But I just knew my faith, and I am a believer in Jesus Christ and that He would protect me. I think they thought I was a little crazed, but I didn't care. I took care of him.

Since we began writing this book, several of those involved have experienced the death of a loved one under hospice care. After a year of diminishing health, Gail's partner, Tom Condon, died in their lake home under Gail's loving care and hospice assistance. Martha's husband, Dr. George Hnatiuk, chose hospice when he was diagnosed with a terminal illness that had progressed beyond treatment options. His life ended in just ten short days, in the same hospital in which he had cared for others for over 40 years. Ann Caulfield-Cook's 101-year-old mother passed away in 2024 after two years in hospice care at home, cared for by her children.

There is no typical hospice patient or end-of-life scenario. In each of these cases, closing the circle was a unique experience that integrated the person's family and relationships, provided comfort measures, and respected the integrity of the person's life.

Experiencing our own family members' deaths can deepen our learning and skills as clinicians. It can help us understand the stress of being the son or daughter, husband or wife, or caregiver of a dying loved one. It can provide us with a roadmap to what may be very meaningful for our patients in their end-of-life journey.

Though spiritual support, palliative care, and hospice care are distinct services, they each help patients "live until they die" by offering patients and their families a path toward closing the circle on their own terms and with as much meaning as possible. Death is a universal experience that leaves no one untouched, but healthcare providers who work in these disciplines can make a tremendous difference in the quality of that ending for both patients and families.

Join our Circle

- In many of our interviews, our colleagues described how their faith or spiritual beliefs help them in their work with end-of-life patients. **What role does your spirituality play in your work with patients and families?**

- Oakwood Hospital had a Spiritual Support Department that helped patients relieve stress, receive guidance or experience closure. **What resources does your hospital or workplace provide to support patients' spiritual needs? How would you approach patients and their families to offer them these resources?**

- Depending on the resources and needs of a hospital, there may be a single palliative care practitioner, or a team of professionals. **Do you have a good understanding of the role of palliative care? How do you explain those services to patients who would benefit from them?**

- In her experience as a social worker, Ann Caulfield-Cook often found that patients had misconceptions about hospice care, believing that it was the withdrawal of all medical care for end-of-life patients. **What misconceptions have you encountered among patients and their families about hospice care at your hospital or workplace? How would you introduce the idea of hospice care and address any misconceptions?**

- Most of the contributors to *Closing the Circle* have had a personal experience with a loved one in hospice. **Have you had a loved one in hospice? If so, has this experience been beneficial in your approach to patients and families under your care?**

Chapter 9

"All Things Considered": Medical Ethics in the Hospital Setting

Ethics is knowing the difference between what you have
a right to do and what is right to do.

—Potter Stewart, Retired Supreme Court Justice of the United States

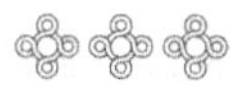

If you are new to the study of medical ethics, this chapter offers an introduction. However, this complex discipline requires time and patience, ongoing formal education, and exposure to ethical issues in the field. It takes years of effort to gain the necessary skills to become proficient in the application of medical ethics, let alone master it.

Since this book is inspired by Gail Daly's career, it is fitting to end with the topic of medical ethics and the hospital's ethics department. Gail recognized the profound importance of ethical standards in the clinical setting, and it informed her work from start to finish, inspiring her to develop procedures for ethical assessment. Though she and her colleagues were successful in raising the profile of medical ethics at Oakwood, they too experienced the same growing pains that any student of ethics encounters on their trip through its learning curve.

While medical ethics is a challenging course of study, it is profoundly worthwhile. We encourage you to continue reading and thinking about this topic because it is an essential tool for addressing the difficult decisions that will always be inherent to healthcare, including the ethical dilemmas you may encounter while providing end-of-life care.

We hope this last chapter will serve as a starting point for your next steps as a student of medical ethics. We also hope that it inspires you to be an advocate for self-determination and a champion for the patient's voice to be heard and followed, just like Gail.

In Chapter 1 we described how Gail and Dr. Haydon formed an ethics process at Oakwood. Their work, in conjunction with the efforts of medical ethicists like Dr. Weber and Dr. Reitemeier, helped raise awareness of patients' rights by applying medical ethics to the fast-paced evolution of life-saving techniques and increasingly complex ethical dilemmas in healthcare.

During that time, Dr. Weber anticipated the emerging ethical dilemmas in the hospital setting:

> In the early 1980s I had my first request to be on an ethics committee. There weren't very many ethics committees at that time. There was just one in the Detroit area that asked me if I would be willing to be on their committee and so that was where it began for me. Then, because myself plus one or two other faculty members were getting requests for participating in discussions and educational programs, we started an Ethics Institute at Mercy College, Detroit, which was my responsibility. Through that we began to work with more hospitals and other healthcare types of organizations. This began in the mid-80s.
>
> It was a timely thing when medical ethics came into the hospitals and the healthcare professions. Long-term care was just starting to be recognized as a serious issue. I had sat in on a talk by a young physician who saw as an issue the ability to keep people alive on mechanical respirators. I remember this because at the time I thought, "Wow, that's an issue that's going to be a biggie," and he agreed. He continued by saying that we could keep people alive this way, but should we?

I was one of the first generation of academic ethicists to move into hospitals. Over the years I have met with over 20 different ethics committees.

Oakwood's blueprint for ethics consultations

There are misconceptions about the role of medical ethics in the hospital, which heightens the need for a required ethics curriculum in all healthcare fields. Ann Caulfield-Cook notes:

> I recently was in the hospital at the bedside of a friend who was dying from cancer and the nurse asked me what I did prior to retirement. I think she figured out I was knowledgeable about end-of-life care. I told her I used to work in the ethics department at a hospital. She commented, "I wish our hospital had an ethics department. We sure need it." The irony is that this conversation took place in an Oakwood satellite hospital where I attended Clinical Ethics Committee meetings.

Every hospital certified by the Joint Commission on Accreditation of Healthcare Organizations (JCAHO) must have a process for addressing ethical dilemmas that arise in the hospital setting. However, that process varies widely. It does not require an ethics committee, and it can involve a team of people or one designated person.

Oakwood had the good fortune of having a full-time ethics staff for the Clinical Ethics Consultation Service (CECS) and a director, Gail, that reported to the multidisciplinary Systems Clinical Ethics Committee (SCEC). Dr. Weber was a contracted employee who reviewed Oakwood's ethics consults and provided ongoing education for the ethics committee members.

Oakwood policy allowed any member of the healthcare team— the bedside nurse, social worker, physician, chaplain, or family member—to request an ethics consultation for a patient. In a hospital setting, most orders for medical care, like diagnostic tests, drugs, and intravenous fluids, are authorized by the physician. Thus, it was remarkable to have a policy that allowed an ethics consult to be initiated by a non-physician and supported by hospital administration and the Medical Staff Office. However, the policy required that the attending physician be notified promptly when a consult had been requested.

Even seasoned staff may feel hesitant to put in an ethics consult request that might risk alienating the medical team. But the feelings of moral distress that come from doing nothing can be far worse. Gail recalled how these feelings often inspired staff to reach out:

> Often nurses would call Family Matters for help, asking for guidance when the family reached an impasse with medical decision-making, or when conflicts between family, staff, or patient occurred. The nurses would feel so frustrated and conflicted, and they automatically called to ask if I would just come over and sit with a family and try to answer something that they had not been able to address.

In many cases, early Family Matters intervention resolved the issue, particularly if it was based on communication challenges. However, the CECS also handled numerous staff-initiated calls, responding in ways that addressed both the issue and any resulting moral distress.

Ethical dilemmas in a medical setting

Ethical dilemmas in a medical setting often involve impasses in determining a patient's legitimate decision-maker, standoffs about whether to withdraw or withhold life-sustaining treatments, clashes of cultural norms, conflicts that delay treatment decisions, or the fair use of scarce resources. A conflict can arise between a patient and family member, among family members themselves, between the legal department and the healthcare provider, or between the family and the medical team.

Though there are many forms of ethical dilemmas, understanding what constitutes an ethical dilemma can help determine whether it is appropriate to seek an ethics consultation. Gail describes the difference in situations that resulted in a Family Matters case and those that prompted the initiation of an ethics consult:

> [T]here were times Family Matters could not resolve an issue by providing supportive communication and family meetings. A formal ethics team was initiated when an impasse was reached or identified as ethical in nature. Some of the hardest cases happened with large families when you needed to find out who was the main decision-maker. Sometimes it was a case in which the decision-maker would say to "do everything," but admitted it was because they didn't want to live with the guilt of withdrawing treatment. I can't tell you how many times I've heard, "I'm not going to be the one to pull the plug."

An ethical dilemma would prompt the questions: What was the right thing to do? What would be the wrong thing? It required an examination from the ethical standards embedded in Western medicine, including honoring self-determination, providing actions that will do good, and avoiding actions that will cause harm.

With each request for an ethics consult, the specifics were presented to the medical ethicist, who would determine if an ethical dilemma truly existed and, if so, identify the ethical principles being challenged. Once this was established, a formal ethics team, which included the ethicist along with four to six members of the SCEC, would participate in the case review. The treating physicians, the patient, family members and friends, and nursing or ancillary staff who were involved with the patient's care were often interviewed as part of the review process. After deliberation, the recommendations were shared with the patient and/or family and medical team and placed in the medical record.

The following ethics case was based on determining the decision-maker for an incapacitated patient in the intensive care unit. The patient was being kept alive on life support despite having no possibility of recovery. The only family member with the authority to grant permission to limit care was a nephew who wasn't responding to attempts to reach him. Dr. Weber describes what took place:

> In this case there was an attorney who had a close relationship with this patient, more as a friend but also as a legal advisor. When the staff asked us what to do, we advised that the next of kin must be considered. But the next of kin was unresponsive after two phone call efforts. Nobody could contact him. However, this attorney was a family friend, and so we got him on a phone call with the medical staff. The people who had requested the ethics consult were also present at the table.
>
> Because it's easier to have one person speak to somebody on the speakerphone, I led the conversation with the attorney. He was able to explain the relationship he had both with the patient and with the nephew. He was asked what he thought the patient would want and he said, based on the patient's whole lifestyle and what he believed in, that the patient would want to be let go [now]. We asked about the nephew, and the attorney said he is not involved and wouldn't have any problem with that decision. Now, that's not very strong, but after the phone call the consultation team members of the ethics committee thought the attorney's information was satisfactory. It's enough information and all we are likely to get, and it fits with what we know about the patient's

previous history.

So, we told the medical staff that we would support terminating life-saving treatment efforts in this case. They were relieved because they were in a quandary about what to do. And they were perfectly satisfied with it too. That would be their medical recommendation as well because his treatment wasn't going anywhere. But they would not have made that decision on their own without our formal recommendation.

I think the role of ethics in this case is that we took charge without stepping out of our bounds. It would have been very easy to say, "Well, we can't reach the next of kin and the friend has no role here." Whether he was an attorney or not was not particularly relevant; he was a friend. What legal would recommend in many cases is that we must keep treating the patient. But this was at a particular hospital which said, "Do the right thing and we'll support you."

There were many ethics consults initiated because of the uncertainty of the rightful or legal decision-maker. State laws dictate a hierarchy of who should serve as an incapacitated patient's decision-maker. The order of authority is as follows: 1) the patient's legally documented healthcare advocate; 2) the designated substitute (surrogate) advocate; 3) a court appointed legal guardian; and, in the absence of any legally appointed agent, 4) the family (DeMartino et al., 2017).

In the majority of cases there is not a legal spokesperson, and a family member must make the medical decisions. If this occurs, state laws also establish a hierarchy of familial relationships. (House Bill 4418 of 2025 - Michigan Legislature, 2025). But relying on what may seem to be a reasonable order of authority can be fraught with problems—for example, if spouses have an antagonistic relationship, or if siblings engage in a power struggle for who is in charge. As we also discussed in Chapter 3, there are many circumstances in which family members question the appropriateness of who should be the decision-maker.

In the absence of a legal advocate, the best case scenario is when there is a consensus among the family regarding who should be the spokesperson, or when decisions are made by family consensus and based on what they think the patient's wishes would be.

The elements of an ethics consult

Principles and purpose

Dr. Weber stresses that the purpose of an ethics consult is not meant to offer a direct solution to a conflict:

> What is an ethics consult? It's not your role to resolve conflicts...It is your role to assess what is going on in a situation and make a recommendation on what good ethical principles say,...about what ethical thinking has to say about how to take the next steps.

> Ethicists are there to sort through the kind of criteria to use...to sort out what is right, or a better decision...or what makes a less better or wrong decision. That's when you need ethics consults.

The field of medical ethics relies, in part, on four well-known principles: autonomy, non-maleficence, beneficence, and justice. Autonomy is respect for a person's authority to make their own decisions, to exercise self-determination. This principle includes the practice of informed consent, truth-telling, and confidentiality. Non-maleficence refers to avoiding harm. Beneficence's goal is to do good, to take the actions that will benefit another's well-being. The principle of justice is to ensure fairness and equity. Beauchamp and Childress (2019) see these principles as fundamental for ethical assessment in the field of medical ethics.

If two or more of these principles conflict, the ethical dilemma can prompt a feeling of moral distress and a desire to find a reasonable resolution. Recommending the "right" thing to do, or at least something better than the worst thing to do, can be challenging.

Gail believes the consistency of the four ethical principles helps to address this challenge:

> It's good that there are ethical principles to think about and go back to. They are like a touchstone. It helps keep the ethics team on track of what principle is at play. Otherwise it can become too individualized, which makes it hard to know what is right in a particular case. Principles gave us parameters to consider.

Dr. Reitemeier's point of view on the purpose of ethics is simple but profound:

> One of the questions I'm asked a fair amount is, "How would you define ethics?" I have a definition that I use that came to me in one sentence in response to that question in a car ride that I remember very distinctly. I thought I nailed it in that one response. It wasn't because I had been mulling it over for a long time, it just happened to be the right question at the right moment. And so, my response is that ethics is the answer to the question: "How ought one live one's life, all things considered?"

"All things considered" is key for a medical ethics recommendation request. Dr. Reitemeier uses a diamond shape to represent the relationship between different options and depict a range of possible actions:

> At the very top of the diamond are the things that you are ethically required to do; these things are mandatory. You cannot operate on someone without informed consent, that sort of thing. The reason these are mandatory is because you can look them up, they are written down.

At the bottom are the things that are forbidden, prohibitive. You cannot kill people. No matter how earnestly they ask, no, that is homicide and against the rules. And again, you know these actions are forbidden because they are written down, you can look it up.

In between is everything that is permitted. Some of what is permitted is a good idea and that is encouraged.... There are other things that are permitted but are discouraged. For example, people will put the trach and PEG [permanent feeding tube] in grandma. It's technically possible, it's permitted within the standard of care, but in my opinion it's a terrible, terrible idea. I'm not willing to do it and I strongly discourage you from asking anybody else to do it. It is permitted but it's a bad idea.

I try to get the physician to see that people do not just come [to them] for interventions, but for the advice about them. We are happy to perform interventions, but we are a little reluctant to give them advice. What people need more than an intervention is our advice about it. And you've got to be able to justify why it is recommended. Don't tell someone he needs a transfusion because his hemoglobin is 5.8. That is not *why* he needs a transfusion.

Dr. Reitemeier's point further supports Dr. Haydon's previous comments in Chapter 2 regarding how a patient or their family will become fixated on improvements in lab results or other tests, but they are often unable to consider that information in the larger context of what is happening: that the patient is not improving overall. This is why it is so important for the physician to use their expertise to advise patients and families about what steps will or will not be effective in the patient's recovery.

The role of policy

One important tool medical ethicists use to identify the criteria relevant to the ethics case and make recommendations is policy.

As with most organizations, healthcare systems have many policies that regulate both administrative and clinical practices. If you are a new hire to a healthcare system, your orientation includes a review of a fraction of these policies. Long-standing employees may be on a committee that reviews and updates policy. Clinical policies are under the auspices of specific departments such as the medical staff, nursing administration, hospital administration, the legal department, or other adjunct clinical areas. Each department is responsible for reviewing and updating their policies.

Oakwood's System Clinical Ethics Committee both provided guidance on hospital policies and was guided by them. Policies drafted by the SCEC included Advance Directives, Determination of Death, End of Life for Adult Patients, and Resolving Conflict When Life-Prolonging Treatment is not Medically Indicated. These policies provide guideposts for decision-making and outlined appropriate action. For example, the Determination of Death policy enumerated all the steps, procedures, and medical disciplines that were required to establish brain death. Thus, if the ethics committee was consulted about a brain death case, they reviewed the Determination of Death policy and cited it in their recommendation. In fact, all written ethics recommendations included references to the pertinent supporting policies.

How important is policy? The following case is a good example of what can take place in a hospital that does not have a policy or guidelines on how to manage non-beneficial treatment. Dr. Weber, who served as ethicist in several hospital systems, describes how, without strong policy, hospital staff would flounder under family demands:

> There was a patient who had been in the hospital for over two years, unresponsive, periodically in intensive care or a step-down unit, and for all this time on life support. He was not involved at all in his own life care decisions. A

son or nephew was a spokesperson and insisted that they, quote, "do everything."

The medical staff had been frustrated by this for a long time but didn't feel that they could resist the family's wishes to continue treatment. This was a hospital in which the legal staff was always warning about going against the family. The chief of staff specifically came to us for advice.

There was no futility policy in the hospital, but a lot of places didn't have them at that time. So, when we got this request, we took it seriously and recognized that what was required was not just feedback on an individual case but the necessity that a policy should be in place. Our thought process was that we needed to establish a policy first and then see how it would apply to this patient. I made a first draft, and we produced more of a statement. It defined non-beneficial treatment as treatment that, regardless of what you did, would not affect the outcome. The statement included that receiving non-beneficial treatment was not a right. What we presented had more developed language, but it was something along those lines. We presented it to the physician and chief of staff.

We were allowed to sit in on the meeting with the family, but the physician was in charge. He told them that this continued treatment wasn't going anywhere, but he wasn't very strong, and the family resisted, and nothing ever came of it. The spokesperson continued to demand care, and so the treatment continued another year. In the end the patient was kept alive for three full years, even though after the first few months there was no medical doubt about what the ultimate outcome was going to be.

When a policy is established, such as one that addresses non-beneficial treatment (futility), its intent is to be equitable, ethical, and universally applicable to individual cases. While the non-beneficial treatment policy did not affect the outcome of the particular patient in the case Dr. Weber describes, its creation defined and codified important decision-making criteria for future patients and families.

For Gail, the importance of well-defined policy was the cornerstone of how the Clinical Ethics Consultation Service and System Clinical Ethics Committee functioned:

> The one way that I think we effectively tried to deal with complex issues was through good policy. We dove into the Brain Death policy and others that related to end-of-life care. Policies really helped us because we could refer to them and that would help guide us. We were not making these tough, spiritual decisions without support. We relied on the careful deliberation of a multi-disciplinary team who applied policy standards and then gave recommendations.

The role of the ethicist

Ethical deliberation requires knowledge, experience, and professionalism. It also requires a specific point of view that is distinct from the role of the healthcare provider. An ethicist's role can bring to light the "shoulds and shouldn'ts" that dictate our actions as a *whole* without getting stuck in the weeds of a particular case. It is the ethicist who helps open our eyes to see beyond a treatment choice or refusal. Dr. Haydon recognized from the beginning of his career that the ethicist's perspective was imperative in the field of healthcare. Gail and her staff would attest to that claim over and over again.

Over the course of his career, Dr. Weber found that the profession evolved due to the successes he and others had in establishing medical ethics as a respected discipline:

I was probably one of the first generation of academic ethicists to start working in hospitals. There were two risks involved in doing that. One is being too self-confident, being the savior: "I know better than you do what is the right thing." The other risk was just the opposite, being too acquiescent in the practices that were established there. After all, these are the medical professionals who know what they are doing, so who am I to say that they should change things? I tried to be somewhere in the middle, trying to be sensitive to both. And it probably was the right thing to do.

At the end of my career, and I don't know if this is because I learned what works or not, I was much more assertive. Taking charge more. Again, my best work in a lot of ways was after I left Oakwood. The reason for that is because I was in a different position. I was an employed ethicist. I had a different standing. And I think that might be the reason I behaved differently because I had different standing. But I was able to do better work as a result. And so, in retrospect, maybe I could have asserted myself earlier, but that's hard to do when you are an outsider.

So, I would say that the lesson learned is that ethics does have a lot to contribute. The last few years I was working I think we made some major changes in a couple different institutions by gaining respect for ethics and then being able to build on that respect.

How do you get that respect? Well, again, I said I was a part of the first generation and so it took a long time. Doing good work, I think, is the bottom line. Knowing what you are talking about. I don't think it's playing politics or trying to please the people who have the power because that power and those people change and then you're out and all that kind of nonsense. But I think it's just being professional.

And so, I guess the lesson to be learned is that ethics must be very professional. I think that applies to efforts to do advanced planning too, with people. It must be very professionally done. Not haphazard. Not following a script but being very professional about thinking through the situation. Recognizing differences that do exist, but taking charge when charge needs to be taken.

Complex cases

Each ethics case at Oakwood had its unique circumstances, which underscores the importance of giving each ethics consult a case-by-case review. Some complex cases involved multiple ethical principles. What may seem at first glance to be a clear-cut scenario of self-determination might be challenged by other ethical considerations.

One such case involved a preemie in the NICU whose parents were Jehovah's Witnesses. They were a young couple and it was their first child. Immediately after birth, the baby required and was given a blood transfusion that saved his life. The NICU doctor initiated an ethics consult because he anticipated the baby would need more blood and wanted the ethics committee to be involved, knowing the parents were torn about giving consent. An ethics consult could provide a level of assurance that medical actions were in line with ethical practice.

Because Oakwood had a long-standing practice of consulting Jehovah's Witness elders to help patients or families when faced with decision-making about receiving blood, the elder joined the formal ethics team meeting, along with the parents and the physician. The parents' spiritual concern and moral distress was caused by their belief that if the baby received another blood transfusion it would "lose a hope for eternal life."

The formal ethics team had to consider both the parents' right to refuse treatment for their child as his legal medical decision-maker (autonomy) and the physician's duty to save the child's life by providing appropriate care (beneficence).

Ethical recommendations must clearly align with ethical principles and support the action that causes least harm, even though other principles can present a parallel track of importance. If there were no other measures that could be taken that could save the baby's life, such as the possible use of non-blood options, then the principles of beneficence (do good) and non-maleficence (do no harm) are influencing the situation. Within this context, the question that needed to be addressed was if the principle of autonomy, which was in the hands of the parents, outweighs the value of saving the life of a minor who could not decide for themself.

It is also not appropriate to coerce people into consenting to something that goes against their beliefs. As Moe Rustom so profoundly explained in Chapter 4, sometimes the decision-maker feels they are being put in the position of "carrying a burden" or "committing a sin." The ethical recommendation was to proceed with giving blood only if it was acutely necessary and obtain permission by court order. In this particular case, the baby was transferred to another hospital and the admitting physician was informed of the medical and ethical dynamics that took place.

Another complex formal ethics case involved a competent patient who had completed an advance directive and designated one of her children as her advocate. After the patient developed dementia, another adult child applied for and was granted legal guardianship from probate court. However, obtaining guardianship of an incompetent adult does not override the authority of the medical advocate or the advance directive a person completed when they were competent. An ethical dilemma arose when the patient's legitimate medical advocate and the newly appointed legal guardian disagreed about the care of their mother. Each claimed to have knowledge of their mother's wishes and the authority to be her decision-maker. The formal ethics team's recommendation was to follow the advance directive document and acknowledge as decision-maker the daughter the patient had previously chosen. Martha recalls the moral distress that both the family and the healthcare team experienced:

> Although the hospital's legal team confirmed the advocate had the right to make the decision to stop medical treatment on the patient, and the formal ethics team also justified the advocate's right to make decisions, the legal guardian was so adamant that their mother would want to be kept alive that the attending physician did not feel comfortable discontinuing life support. The attending did make the patient a DNR, but because of the enormous pushback from the guardian to continue life support and threatened legal measures, the treatment that was keeping the patient alive was continued.

> This standoff between family members overshadowed the patient's right to self-determination and caused moral distress for the advocate. The advocate knew it was her duty to follow the wishes of her mother, who did not want extraordinary measures taken or to live a marginal existence on life support. It also distressed the nursing staff who continued administering treatments that were prolonging the patient's death. This scenario lasted for many days until, still on the ventilator, the patient finally expired.

> When it became apparent the patient's death was imminent, all the family members were notified but only the daughter who was the advocate came to be with her mother. Gail and I were also at the bedside. I clearly remember that on that grey Michigan day, a sunstream entered from a window and flooded the bed just as the patient's heart stopped beating. That ray of light was a bit

of solace, a spiritual thing, as Gail would say. But it came after a long battle between siblings that prolonged the patient's suffering and unfortunately fell into the category of an ugly death.

In this case, the ethics recommendation to acknowledge the advocate as the medical decision-maker was based on the "right thing to do," but a formal ethics consult recommendation does not carry the same clout as medical orders and is not always followed by the healthcare provider.

How likely is it that the attending physician will follow those recommendations? In Gail's experience it depended upon the physician:

> When the physicians requested our help, they often wanted either confirmation that they were moving in the right direction or to see if they might have missed something. We would just chime in together as a team.

> But there were also physicians who did not want ethics involved at all. It was like they were afraid of us. I remember one time a physician referred to us as "the ethics police." But that wasn't true. I tried to convey that we were specifically there to help the physicians and their patients and the family, and to make sure there was adequate communication and all the facts they needed to make a good decision.

But it is still the role of clinical ethics to illuminate the ethical perspective and the reasons why following those recommendations serves the better good or at least causes less harm.

When ethical considerations clash

Ethical issues also arise when patients refuse medical recommendations. This became evident in the landmark case of

Dax (Donald) Cowart, who at the age of 25, suffered horrific burns over 65% of his head and body from a propane gas explosion (Gerrek, 2018). The accident left him blind and disabled. Most of his fingers needed to be amputated. He experienced extreme pain throughout the 14 months of treatments and never relented in his demands for them to stop. Although he was deemed competent, his mother kept granting consent and his twice-daily treatments were continued. This case highlights what can take place when both legal and ethical applications of self-determination are not followed and the patient's wishes are disregarded.[4] Dr. Reitemeier adds:

> Dax Cowart said to his dying day that he had been violated, and it should never have been allowed. The fact that he had a successful law career, an import/export business and became a millionaire was irrelevant. He claimed even though he now had a good life and didn't want to die, it was irrelevant in regard to the unwanted treatment he was forced to endure.

Gail had an opportunity to meet with Dax:

> I was able to attend an ethics lecture given by Dax at Michigan State University. Through tremendous fortitude on his part, he became a lawyer and a national speaker for patient's rights. There was an opportunity for me to meet him after the lecture. He was in a wheelchair and extended the stub of his arm to me, which I shook. The burns had reduced both arms to mere stubs. I will never forget him or his story.

In another case, Dr. Reitemeier recounted an occasion when a woman needed an extensive surgical procedure, but rejected this

---

4   *For more information on this case, see the Resources section at the end of the book.*

treatment because she was terrified of being touched. She refused the surgery and stopped eating:

> Psychiatry weighed in and said she couldn't make decisions because she was not competent. She has lost her autonomy. This is the great principle that everybody thinks the ethical alphabet begins with, "A is for autonomy," and it's not true. If you read all eight editions of the *Principles of Biomedical Ethics* they say over and over and over, no, autonomy is not the big one. She doesn't have any autonomy, but she still retains her sovereignty, the ownership of her body and the right to control what happens to it, and that it is not violated as she sees it. She was enrolled in hospice and allowed to die. We could medically imprison and enforce treatment, but to what end?

Dr. Reitemeier expanded on how sovereignty differs from autonomy:

> Sovereignty is the ethical right to control what happens to your person while you are alive and after you are dead. Otherwise it's called mutilation of a corpse. Otherwise it's called disrespecting the intent of the deceased.
>
> And the government has an entire division called Decedent Affairs. How you take care of the interest of dead bodies. The whole point of a will, what do I do with my money and my property, is to respect me in the future when I am not here anymore. It's a legal obligation to do that grounded in the ethics of respect for sovereignty, not autonomy, but sovereignty: the right to control what is yours. And there is nothing more yours than your body. Even if you can't do it rationally, if what other people want to do with your body you understand and you object, that should be protected unless it harms others.

This level of distinction and nuance is a reminder that medical ethics and ethical deliberation requires the expertise of those who are educated in the field to make sure every potential option and outcome is assessed. The distinction that Dr. Reitemeier made above plays a role in many cases that involve a patient's refusal to accept a recommended treatment for a curable injury or illness: patients who refuse a life-saving measure that requires an appendage be amputated, or, in the previously described case, when a patient refuses the PEG tube.

Although Gail was passionate in her efforts to fight for a person's right to choose, she found that she struggled most with cases where those choices disregarded medical inevitability:

> It was all the different cases of futility, or what is more currently recognized as non-beneficial treatment. In those cases multiple specialists came in and assessed the patient and made the diagnosis and prognosis that there was nothing more they could medically offer. Then in comes the family and demands the physician continue with everything.

> Most of those cases were really rough. We would sit down and have an in-depth meeting with all the doctors and family. We would cram into the conference room and first make sure everybody understood what the medical diagnosis was and what it means, the likelihood of the outcomes and the futility of the case. We would discuss if there was any hope of recovery at all.

> Some physicians were comfortable saying that they had nothing more to offer. But there were other physicians that would say there were other things to try, even knowing in their heart of hearts it really was not going to make a difference.

> In this scenario the formal ethics team would often recommend that non-beneficial treatment did not have to be offered or continued. The formal recommendation,

which also included the circumstances of the case along with the team's ethical deliberations and reasoning, would be entered in the medical chart. But an ethics recommendation was not a medical order. It was up to the treating physician to decide how to proceed.

Being part of an ethics consultation can involve many variables, and often ethical principles can seem to be at odds with each other. Dr. Weber states that the key is to discern, in each case at hand, what is the right thing to do, and how you determine what is right. He says, "Right is the term I would prefer. What is *right*, rather than the term *ethical*." He elaborates:

> There are two different "right things" in medical ethics: one is the right thing for those who are providing the care, and one is the right thing for those who are receiving the care. And they're very different. A lot of times people confuse those.

He clarifies:

> What is right for those who receive the care often involves value considerations that vary somewhat from the professional's judgment about the standards of good healthcare— anything from asserting the right to decline unwanted healthcare to a desire to try something more even when judged medically "futile" by physicians.

Take for example the case in which a blood transfusion could save a life but goes against the strongly held beliefs of the patient, or the person with dementia who does not want their foot amputated, or the brain dead patient whose family will not allow the removal of life support. All the potential resolutions of these cases hinge both on an understanding of what the healthcare provider is trying to achieve, and on what the patient and/or family understands or is willing to accept. Both perspectives require ethical consideration often in the face of moral distress felt by the family, the staff, and even the ethics consultation team. In the complexity of modern healthcare, we always come back to the same question: what is the right thing to do? Often the answer is not absolute, but rather, it is the choice that does the most good and the least harm.

The value of medical ethics

The application of medical ethics is challenging for new healthcare providers, and continues to be challenging even for seasoned medical professionals. Ethical interventions are not always perceived as beneficial and are sometimes even seen as antagonistic by practitioners, but they are always meant to provide crucial structure to difficult decisions. In the myriad of circumstances that can confound medical decision-making, applied medical ethics establishes standards to follow.

Join our Circle

- The System Clinical Ethics Committee and the Clinical Ethics Consultation Service at Oakwood responded to ethics consultation requests throughout Oakwood's system and offered recommendations for ethical dilemmas. **What resources, processes, or services related to medical ethics does your institution offer? How accessible do you think these resources and services are?**

- Dr. Weber and Chris Westphal expressed how the advancement of medical treatments have blurred the line between saving a life and prolonging the dying process. **What developing technologies or treatments do you think will complicate decision-making around when to withdraw life support when there is no hope of recovery?**

- Gail describes the difference between asking for FMSS to intervene by talking with family and staff and actually making a request for an ethics consult. **What criteria would you use to determine if a formal ethics consult is warranted? Do you have staff at your hospital to discuss ethics concerns before requesting an ethics consultation?**

- Even though Oakwood had a policy and procedure for initiating an ethics consult, staff were often hesitant to do so, fearing they might be perceived as criticizing a provider's handling of a patient's care. **Have you ever experienced "moral distress" in deciding whether to raise your ethics concerns? Are there times you wish you would have done something more, but were wary of the backlash it would cause?**

Chapter 10

Full Circle

Not to transmit an experience is to betray it.

—Elie Wiesel

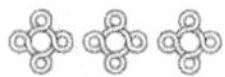

The hard work of Gail, Dr. Haydon, Chris Westphal, Dr. Weber, and the other dynamic professionals that served on the System Clinical Ethics Committee created a truly remarkable program that elevated the practice of medical ethics at Oakwood. It achieved this goal by collaborating with the medical staff, administration, and many ancillary departments. There were also coordinated efforts between satellite hospitals, and participation with universities and established medical ethics affiliations (Michigan State University, American Society of Humanities and Bioethics, Medical Ethics Resource Network of Michigan).

From the beginning of Gail's professional career, she took on the responsibility of making a positive impact on the healthcare experience. Even in her twilight years she continues to reach out through her participation in *Closing the Circle*, sharing the lessons she and others have learned throughout their careers. Although this book captures the fundamentals of the wisdom she accrued over her lifetime of service to others, all the personal experiences and the trials and the growing pains that were part of her everyday journey cannot adequately be depicted here. With each day, each patient, and each family's sorrow, anger, or grief, she committed herself to "doing the right thing…all things considered." It could weigh heavy on the heart, but she kept moving forward, and she taught those around her how to do the same. All things considered, it made a difference.

When Gail was asked about her legacy and what she would like to be remembered for, she said:

> In terms of a legacy, I don't see myself as being important enough for that word. But I've always identified my wishes with a story. You may have heard this story. It is about a little boy walking along the ocean shore. The tide had gone out and there were just hundreds of starfish that were stranded on the beach. When the sun hit them, they looked iridescent. Even though they were scattered all over the little boy was frantically throwing them, one by one, back into the ocean. An older man came by and asked him, "Son, what are you trying to do? Look at all these starfish! How can you possibly make a difference?" But the boy picked up another one and threw it back in the water and replied, "I made a difference for that one."

That says it all. If you can make a difference for even one person, it feels good. It's the right thing.

References

Adashi, E. Y., Walters, L. B., & Menikoff, J. A. (2018). The Belmont Report at 40: Reckoning With Time. *American Journal of Public Health*, *108*(10), 1345–1348. https://doi.org/10.2105/ajph.2018.304580

Barbret, L. C., Westphal, C. G., & Daly, G. A. (1997). Meeting Information Needs of Families of Critical Care Patients. *Journal for Healthcare Quality*, *19*(2), 5–10. https://doi.org/10.1111/j.1945-1474.1997.tb01173.x

Beauchamp, T. L., & Childress, J. F. (2019). *Principles of Biomedical Ethics* (8th ed.). Oxford University Press.

Curtis, J, Patrick, D, Shannon, S, Treece, P, Engelberg, R & Rubenfeld, G. (2001). The family conference as a focus to improve communication about end-of-life care in the intensive care unit: Opportunities for improvement. *Critical Care Medicine*, *29*(2), N26-N33.

DeMartino, E. S., Dudzinski, D. M., Doyle, C. K., Sperry, B. P., Gregory, S. E., Siegler, M., Sulmasy, D. P., Mueller, P. S., & Kramer, D. B. (2017). Who Decides When a Patient Can't? Statutes on Alternate Decision Makers. *New England Journal of Medicine*, *376*(15), 1478–1482. https://doi.org/10.1056/nejmms1611497

Emanuel, L. L. (1989). The Medical Directive. *JAMA*, *261*(22), 3288. https://doi.org/10.1001/jama.1989.03420220102036

Epstein, R. M., & Street, R. L. (2011). Shared Mind: Communication, Decision Making, and Autonomy in Serious Illness. *The Annals of Family Medicine*, *9*(5), 454–461. https://doi.org/10.1370/afm.1301

Foster, L. W., & McLellan, L. J. (2002). Translating Psychosocial Insight into Ethical Discussions Supportive of Families in End-of-Life Decision-Making. *Social Work in Health Care, 35*(3), 37–51. https://doi.org/10.1300/j010v35n03_03

Gerrek, M. (2018). Getting Past Dax. *AMA Journal of Ethics, 20*(6), 581–588. https://doi.org/10.1001 journalofethics.2018.20.6.mhst1-1806

Holmes, O. W. (1892). *Medical essays 1842-1882* (Vol. 9). Houghton, Mifflin.

House Bill 4418 of 2025 - Michigan Legislature. (2025). Mi.gov. https://www.legislature.mi.gov/Bills/ Bill?ObjectName=2025-HB-4418

Jaworska, A. (2009, March 24). *Advance Directives and Substitute Decision-Making.* Illc.uva.nl. https://seop.illc.uva.nl/entries/advance-directives/

Levin, S. M. (1990, July 2). *H.R.4449 - 101st Congress (1989-1990): Patient Self Determination Act of 1990.* www.congress.gov. https://www.congress.gov/bill/101st-congress/ house-bill/4449

Patterson, K., Grenny, J., Mcmillan, R., & Switzler, A. (2012). *Crucial conversations: Tools for talking when stakes are high.* New York Mcgraw-Hill Professional.

Puchalski, C. M., Epstein, L. C., Fox, E., Johnston, M. A., Kallenberg, G. A., Kitchens, L. W., Larson, D. B., Lu, F. G., McLaughlin, M. A., O'Donnell, J. F., Sarraf, K., Swyers, J. P., Woolliscroft, J., & Anderson, M. B. (1999). Report

III Contemporary issues in medicine: Communication in medicine. *Medical School Objectives Project.*

Quinn, J. R., Schmitt, M., Baggs, J. G., Norton, S. A., Dombeck, M. T., & Sellers, C. R. (2012). Family Members' Informal Roles in End-of-Life Decision Making in Adult Intensive Care Units. *American Journal of Critical Care*, *21*(1), 43–51. https://doi.org/10.4037/ajcc2012520

Worden, J. W. (2018). *Grief counseling and grief therapy: A handbook for the mental health practitioner* (5th ed.). Springer Publishing Company, Llc.

Resources

The wide range of topics that are included in *Closing the Circle* are only entry points for your study of the many facets of end-of-life care. We hope that these pages will offer you a better understanding of these topics, empower you to improve your practice in the clinical setting, and encourage a deeper dive into your areas of interest. The following resources provide supplementary information for further study and reflection.

If you would like to contact the authors or contributors of *Closing the Circle*, we can be reached at closingthecirclegma@gmail.com. We appreciate your feedback.

Chapter 6—Understanding the Connection: Communicating with Patients and Family

Bernacki, R. E., & Block, S. D. (2014). Communication about serious illness care goals: a review and synthesis of best practices. *JAMA internal medicine, 174*(12), 1994-2003.

Moss, A. (n.d.). *The Ask-Tell-Ask Approach to Conversations with Seriously Ill Patients**.

https://wvendoflife.org/media/1190/ask-tell-ask-2019.pdf

Alvin Moss draws from Rachelle Bernacki and Susan Block's article to provide an example of the Ask-Tell-Ask method of communication. The method was aimed at achieving sustainable clinical outcomes by ensuring patient understanding of information as it was being provided to them.

Chapter 7—Advance Directives

My Voice - My Choice

Daly, G., Westphal, C., Felt, J.K. (2011) *My Voice - My Choice* (Publication No. J117712) Rev. 2/11. Copyright 2006 Oakwood Healthcare System

The *My Voice - My Choice* advance directive document, originally produced in 2003, was reprinted many times. It was revised in 2011 and again in 2014. Thousands of copies were distributed and provided without charge throughout the hospital system, in physicians' offices and in countless educational sessions held throughout Southeast Michigan and beyond. Its original version contained inserts with questions to prompt conversations and information explaining medical terms and treatments a critically ill patient may need. Later versions incorporated the information into the booklet itself.

My Voice - My Choice is no longer in print. If you would like a digital copy of the 2011 document, it can be obtained upon request by emailing the authors at: closingthecirclegma@gmail.com

Nancy Cruzan

Colby, W. H. (2002). *Long Goodbye: The Deaths of Nancy Cruzan.* Hay House Inc.

Taub, S. (2001). "Departed, Jan 11, 1983; At Peace, Dec 26, 1990." *AMA Journal of Ethics, 3*(7).

https://doi.org/10.1001
virtualmentor.2001.3.7.imhl1-0107

These two resources offer a fuller version of the Nancy Cruzan case. William H. Colby was the attorney for the Cruzan family.

His book is an account of the personal and legal history of Nancy Cruzan and her family. Sara Taub also provides the history of the Cruzan's long struggle to be at peace with their daughter's death.

Additional resources for advance medical directives

Aging with Dignity. (n.d.). Aging with Dignity. https://agingwithdignity.org

> Aging with Dignity is a non-profit organization that defends the rights of all people as they approach the end of life. Their Five Wishes advance care planning program has helped bring peace and comfort to over 43 million families.

CaringInfo: Resources for serious illness and end-of-life care decision-making and caregiving. (n.d.). CaringInfo. https://www.caringinfo.org

> This program from the National Alliance for Care at Home provides information, guides, and resources related to advance directives, palliative care, and hospice care. On the website's advance directive page, you can download advance directive forms by state.

Durable Power of Attorney for Health Care. (n.d.). www.michigan.gov.

https://www.michigan.gov/fyit/health/durable-power-of-attorney-for-health-care

> The State of Michigan's website has links to Power of Attorney forms. Enter "advance directive" in the search field and you will be directed to the page "Power of Attorney and Advance Directive Resources." Every state should have a resource. Please note that not every state will have a standard

online form because state laws vary. It is important that you complete a form that will be legally recognized in the state where you reside.

Have You Had The Conversation? - The Conversation Project. (2019). The Conversation Project. https://theconversationproject.org

The Conversation Project is a public engagement initiative of the Institute for Healthcare Improvement (IHI). Its goal is to help everyone talk about their wishes for care through the end of life so that those wishes can be understood and respected. The home page has links to several guides, such as "Guide to Being a Health Care Proxy," "Guide to choosing a Health care Proxy," and a "Conversation Starter Guide."

Chapter 8—Spiritual Support, Palliative Care and Hospice Care: Paths Toward Comfort and Meaning

American Academy of Hospice and Palliative Medicine. (n.d.). Aahpm.org. https://aahpm.org

AAHPM is the professional organization for physicians, nurses, and other healthcare providers who specialize in hospice and palliative medicine. It focuses on training, resources, networking, and advocacy to advance hospice and palliative medicine and improve the care of patients with serious illness.

Homepage - National Alliance for Care at Home. (2024, September 4). National Alliance for Care at Home. https://allianceforcareathome.org/

The National Association for Home Care & Hospice (NAHC) and the National Hospice and Palliative Care Organization (NHPCO) have come together to form the National Alliance for Care at Home (the Alliance). The Alliance is the largest organization representing, advocating for, educating, and connecting providers of care in the home for millions of patients across the US.

Chapter 9—Medical Ethics

Kliever, L. D. (Ed.) (1989). *Dax's Case. Essays in Medical Ethics and Human Meaning.* Southern Methodist University Press.

Hillard Law. (2025, March 19). *Dax Cowart - 20/20 Monday with Charles Gibson.* [Video].

YouTube. https://www.youtube.com watch?v=R29rU5KIqfw

Parsi, K., & Winslade, W. J. (2019). Why Dax's Case Still Matters. *The American Journal of Bioethics*, *19*(9), 8–10. https://doi.org/10.1080/15265161.2019.1643944

These resources give more information about the case of Dax Cowart. Lonnie Kliever presents an edited group of essays on the medical and moral issues that arose from Dax's experience. Kayhan Parsi and William Winslade provide an overview of the case and cite additional resources and films. The 20/20 segment related to the case available on YouTube offers a powerful look at Dax's story.

Acknowledgements

Gail Daly

I would first like to acknowledge Tom Condon, my life partner of 40 years, who supported and grounded my life. He continued to support me throughout our many years together and was always interested in the work I did. He even came up with the slogan, "You better use your voice before you lose your choice"—the tagline for the *My Voice - My Choice* advance directive document produced at Oakwood. My daughters Wendy and Tammy have been part of this lifelong journey as well and have helped me to better understand how family can influence our decision-making.

Dr. Paul Haydon must also be mentioned. Paul and I spent many professional years together and it was because of his fortitude and determination that the medical staff agreed to address clinical ethics in a formalized way. Because of Paul's influence he was able to push through barriers and he participated from day one in getting things going.

There were countless other people who supported my work, who listened to and understood my vision and helped it come to fruition. I am grateful for all of them. Certain people who were particularly influential I would like to mention.

Christine Westphal and I first worked together in Oakwood's cardiac critical care unit…She shared the same vision that I did: to include family in patient care. She became an integral part of advancing the concept of family-centered care into the Family Matters model. Chris's influence is visible in the pages of this book. She was known for her ability to make things happen and has always been known as a valuable resource and lifelong learner.

Within the Family Matters realm, I want to mention Moe Rustom, Martha Hnatiuk, Don Johnson, Pat Abele, and Patricia Barker Groves, all who made such important contributions to our service and to the patients and families they guided and provided with compassionate attention. I am very thankful for their outstanding dedication in the roles that they played as Family Matters staff on the units and as members of the System Clinical Ethics Committee. Don's role in developing policy was particularly valuable. Mary Catherine Wright, Clinical Nurse Specialist, was our Family Matters counterpart at Heritage Hospital, a satellite of the Oakwood Healthcare System. She had the special challenge of running Family Matters solo and became an indispensable person to the patients she served.

Ann Caulfield-Cook, PhD, took over the role as supervisor of the Clinical Ethics Consultation Service after I retired, and she was the right person for me to pass on my baton. Ann took on the challenge with grace and skill. Eileen Dunleavy, RN, was part of the ethics consultation service at that time and stayed the course until her recent retirement. I am grateful for both of them and their efforts to sustain the program that started so many years ago.

The Clinical Ethics Committee was made up of an assortment of disciplines representing people that served with dedication and knowledge to advance the practice of ethical standards and serve as a resource to staff. It was a multidisciplinary powerhouse of tremendously talented people such as Jan Sladewski, Chaplain Beverly Beltramo, the indispensable Dr. Leonard Weber and notable Dr. Paul Reitemeier, Kay Felt, Joanne Lax, Eide Alawan, and many others who represented social work, medicine, administration, spiritual support, and the community at large.

I would also like to acknowledge the physicians who were willing to work alongside us and who recognized the value we could and did bring to the table each day, the nurses who called on us when they recognized special attention was needed, and all the ancillary staff from various departments. Because of their collaboration, we were better equipped to navigate how to help our patients and support their family members.

Many thanks to Ann Caulfield-Cook and Martha Hnatiuk, who collaborated on writing *Closing the Circle*, and to Dana Dunham, whose editing skill and attention to detail was essential for this project. All of their efforts are very much appreciated. Thank you to those who provided their valuable feedback during the whole process: Leonard Weber, Joanne Lax, Chris Westphal, Moe Rustom, and others. The process of completing *Closing the Circle* was certainly a journey, but we made it through because of everyone who supported us.

Finally, thank you to my colleagues who allowed us to interview them and share the lessons they learned. It is my hope that these precious experiences will not be lost. May they be used as a guide in the art of compassionate care, communicative care, and ethical end-of-life care.

Ann Caulfield-Cook

First, I want to thank Gail and Martha for inviting me in on their project. When they invited me to lunch and presented the idea to me, I was surprised. They already had an outline for the book and completed all the interviews with their colleagues. Martha gave me the transcripts of the interviews and suggested I read them to help me decide. I enjoyed reading the interviews of our Oakwood colleagues. Between working with two of my favorite friends and working with outstanding interview material, I could not say no. It has been an exciting journey with them. And I want to thank the interviewees for sharing their personal stories that are a critical contribution to the book. As a clinical social worker, I have years of confidentially listening to personal stories of brave individuals of both a heartwarming and tragic nature. The interviewees opened up to Gail and Martha at the intimate kitchen table setting. They trustingly shared their stories with Gail and Martha, and we aimed to respect their sharing in this book.

I must acknowledge my family's support through this journey: my husband Mike, and my siblings Mary, Matt, and Mike. My family has been my greatest source of support and encouragement in this venture. My parents, Richard and Ceal, promoted education and reading in our childhood and would be pleased with my work on this book. My mother was alive during a majority of this project but declining due to dementia. She died about a year before we finished the editing of the book. The experience of helping her in closing her circle was a profound lesson in love and respect for her end-of-life wishes.

I want to thank our readers who gave us feedback during the writing of the book. My sister, Mary, was one of our initial readers. My good friend and retired nurse, Bonie, was also a reader and gave us needed praise at a critical period. Another reader was my daughter-in-law Kate, an Assistant Professor at Chamberlain University's nursing program. We gave her the first half of the book to read, and she was very encouraging. She gave us helpful suggestions. Thank you, Kate. And my cousin Dan Riney, an editor, was our first editor who corrected our egregious errors in grammar, punctuation, and spelling. I relearned the fundamentals of grammar again from him.

Lastly, I want to mention Martha's husband, George. He thanked me for taking on the project and helping Martha one day while we were out on our boat. He was a presence in the home when I worked with Martha and is greatly missed. The work at Oakwood Clinical Ethics Department was one of those rare supportive and loving work environments that led to forming bonds with these two women and others including Eileen, Joanne, Jan, Mary Catherine,

Pete Zingas (an attorney who did our guardianships cases), and many more employees that I interacted with over the years.

Martha Hnatiuk

I would like to acknowledge my late husband, Dr. George Hnatiuk, whom I adored and who supported and encouraged me in whatever I chose to pursue. It was George who had the idea to introduce me to Gail Daly, because he knew I was interested in clinical ethics and that I wanted to be back in a hospital setting.

That introduction to Gail led to my seat as a community member on Oakwood's ethics committee and then staff member for Family Matters and the Clinical Ethics Consultation Service. It also led to a friendship with Gail that I treasure, and many profound interactions with other staff members, hospital employees, patients, and families. Under Gail's guidance I had the privilege of entering the sacred space that occurs at end of life.

I am deeply grateful to those who helped me learn how to navigate closing the circle: Gail, Chris Westphal, Moe Rustom, Don Johnson, Pat Abele, and of course Leonard Weber. They played an important part in compassionately allowing me to self-critique and mature into a role that became for me, undoubtedly, remarkable beyond description.

Thank you to all those whom we interviewed. Your honest accounts are just a glimpse of what took place on a daily basis and are the backbone of the message we hope to convey.

It was Gail's wish that these stories be shared. The accounts within this book only skim the surface of what occurred. Trying to convey the importance of the healthcare provider's role through stories and lessons was incredibly challenging, but their lessons are too important to lose, and so this is our attempt to bring the value of others' experiences to you.

I also want to thank my children who supported my efforts along the way, and especially Anna Dewey, who became another set of eyes to help review the project. Finally, there are two very important people I want to acknowledge. First, I want to thank co-author Ann Caulfield-Cook, who steadfastly guided, contributed, cajoled, and managed the project every step of the way. She is the primary reason that a promise I made to Gail to capture and share these experiences made it to the finish line. Second, I want to thank our editor Dana Dunham, who took the thoughts we were trying so hard to convey, polished and refined them, wove them together in a seamless way, and skillfully closed the circle on this project. I hope all of our combined efforts will make a difference in your own practice and in the delivery of healthcare.

Closing the Circle
Participant Profiles

Derek Bair, MD, FAAP

Dr. Bair began his practice as a Neonatologist at Oakwood Hospital in Dearborn, Michigan, in 1994 after a short time in academic medicine at Tufts University School of Medicine in Boston, Massachusetts. He is currently the Regional Director of Neonatology at Corewell Health East, comprised of seven delivering hospitals and three level 3 NICUs. Dr. Bair attended Wright State University School of Medicine, did his pediatric internship and residency at the Medical College of Ohio and fellowship at Baylor College of Medicine specializing in Neonatal and Perinatal Medicine. His expertise is in congenital abnormalities, congenital heart disease, premature infants, newborn screening, and high-risk deliveries.

Gail Daly, PhD, MSA, RN

As the driving force behind *Closing the Circle*, many of Gail's professional accomplishments are highlighted in the first chapter. A life-long student, after attaining a BSN she went on to receive her master's degree in health services administration from Central Michigan and a PhD in Interdisciplinary Studies from America/ Capella University. Gail was employed at Oakwood Hospital, Dearborn from 1989 until 2012. Her positions ranged from the emergency room to critical care nurse to nurse manager to co-founder and director of Family Matters Support Service and the Clinical Ethics Center. She was the recipient of numerous awards and honors including a "local hero" award which recognized excellence in nursing, the Michigan Business & Professional Association Professional/Leadership Award, American Association of critical care nurses Inno Vision Award, and recognized by the Governor of Michigan's End-of-Life Commission for the *My Voice - My Choice* advance care packet, cited as Best Practice. She had many professional affiliations, numerous journal publications and was tireless in presenting information about advance directives throughout metro-Detroit and beyond. Her capacity and skill to serve as a manager, administrator, innovator and educator never overshadowed her dedication as a nurse and her insistence on being called Gail throughout her career.

Eileen Dunleavy, BSN, RN

Eileen Dunleavy is a retired Corewell Health ICU nurse, CEC consultant and Ethics Committee member. She has a BSN from Madonna College and is certified in ethics consultation by the American Society of Bioethics and Humanities. She served on the Gift of Life committee during her career at Legacy Oakwood and Corewell Health. She was responsible for receiving and conducting requests for ethics consultations, executing consultations including expert analysis and following up with cases. Her role also included participation in hospital rounds proactively identifying ethical conflicts and educating providers on best practices for dealing with ethical conflicts in patient care.

Paul Haydon, MD, FACP, FCCP

Dr. Haydon worked for many years as an intensivist at Corewell (formerly Oakwood) Health in Dearborn, Michigan. He received his medical degree from Michigan State University College of Human Medicine and is certified in critical care and internal medicine from the American Board of Internal Medicine. He was a member of the group practice, Critical Care Medicine Associates. He was instrumental in the advancement of ethical standards of care at Oakwood, the first physician member of

Oakwood's Clinical Ethics Committee and its first chair. It was Dr. Haydon who coined the phrase 'Family Matters' while working with Gail Daly and Chris Westphal in critical care, recognizing the role family played in the delivery of comprehensive healthcare. He began practicing medicine at Oakwood in 1983 and retired from Corewell Health in 2025.

George Hnatiuk, MD

Dr. Hnatiuk was an internist and hematologist with a private practice in Dearborn Michigan that spanned 40 years. In addition to his work with patients he had numerous administrative roles, including six years as Oakwood's Chief of Staff. He was also actively involved in the hospital's Cancer Center and instrumental in achieving credentialing for the Cancer Program. As Chairman of the Cancer Committee, he was the longest-serving chair of any committee at the hospital. He was recognized twice as Teacher of the Year by the hospital's Residency program, Dr. Hnatiuk studied medicine at the University of Innsbruck, did his internship and residency at Oakwood hospital and hematology fellowship at Henry Ford Hospital, Detroit. He is the late husband of Martha Hnatiuk and was a firm supporter of CTC. He strongly advocated that the stories and lessons which took place under Gail's tenure be shared.

Joanne Lax, JD

Joanne Lax is a retired health law attorney. During her forty years of practice, she advised healthcare organizations on many clinical ethics issues. These included end-of-life care and advance care planning; rights of mentally incapacitated and disabled patients and the provider's responsibilities to them; standards for surrogate healthcare decision-making; clinical research using embryos; allocation of resources in times of shortage or emergency; religious objections to healthcare – particularly for minors; and ethics committee policies and procedures. Joanne served as a member of and co-chair of the Clinical Ethics Committee at Oakwood and then Beaumont Hospital and as a member of the Clinical Ethics Committee at Legacy Beaumont-Royal Oak Hospital. She assisted in updating a version of *My Voice - My Choice* and participated in Clinical Ethics Committee case consultations. She was a frequent presenter on clinical ethics issues at a variety of professional conferences.

Father Richard Leliaert, PhD

Father Leliaert is a priest of the Archdiocese of Detroit. Currently retired, he has served as a priest for 53 years in three main capacities: as a college professor of Religious Studies, mainly at Nazareth College in Kalamazoo (1977-1987); as a healthcare chaplain and Manager of Spiritual Support Services, mainly at Oakwood Hospital in Dearborn, MI (1992-2006); and as a pastor of St. Robert Bellarmine Parish in Redford (2006-2018).

Father Richard was Co-chair of the Oakwood Healthcare System's corporate Ethics Committee and served on the Clinical Ethics Committee. He was a member of the Transcultural Strategic Committee (with special focus on Muslim and Hispanic populations), the Parish Nursing Advisory Board, and board president of the National Association of Catholic Chaplains. In addition to conducting lectures and workshops on ethical issues he published articles in various journals on grief and bereavement and end of life issues. Fr. Leliaert received his Doctorate from the Graduate Theological Union and the University of California at Berkeley.

Tony Shomari Marshall DMin, BCC, ACPE CE

Rev. Marshall is a Board-Certified chaplain with the Association of Professional Chaplains and a Certified Educator with the Association of Clinical Pastoral Education. He is a consecrated Bishop and ordained Pastor in the Pentecostal Christian Church. He has been a chaplain for nearly 30 years and an educator for 15 years. During that time, he has taught and trained hundreds of professional chaplains and ministers of all faith traditions. Being a former college professor, Tony has written several books on spiritual formation, and he travels extensively lecturing and speaking on spirituality, trauma, and healthcare in universities, hospitals, churches, and community organizations. For the past 9 years Tony has served as the Program Manager of the Clinical Pastoral Education Center at Michigan Medicine, The University of Michigan Hospital in Ann Arbor.

Jacqueline Reitemeier-Mohs, MD

Dr. Reitemeier-Mohs is a physician in South-East Michigan. She received her medical degree from Michigan State University College of Human Medicine and is certified in internal, geriatric and palliative medicine from the American Board of Internal Medicine. She has held Medical Director positions in multiple service lines, including Geriatric and Palliative Medicine, Hospice and Clinical Ethics. She is committed to equity and compassion in care. During her tenure at Oakwood Hospital, Dearborn, she served as the co-chair of the System Clinical Ethics Committee for 8 years, then as a clinical ethics consultant and physician advisor to the Beaumont Health System Clinical Ethics Consultation Service. She has conducted hundreds of clinical ethics case consultations and contributed to the development of clinical ethics policies.

Paul Reitemeier, PhD

Paul Reitemeier is a retired philosopher who worked for more than three decades in health centers, intensive care units and university philosophy classrooms across the midwest in Michigan, Wisconsin, Minnesota, and Nebraska. He also worked in government on the National Ethics Committee as senior clinical ethicist and Communications Chief at the National Center for Ethics in the Veterans Administration in Washington, D.C. Paul holds a BA in Philosophy from the University of Kansas (1984), a master's degree in Medical Ethics from the University of Kansas, and a PhD in Philosophy, concentration in bioethics, from Michigan State University (1992). He performed more than 2 thousand clinical case consultations, collaborated on VHA position papers on gifts to clinicians from the pharmaceutical industry, and developed an ICU early warning system for ethics consultation requests. He has published many articles, book chapters and encyclopedia entries on a variety of topics.

Moe Rustom, MSA, RN, FACHE

Moe has over 30 years' healthcare experience in the clinical and management field and has been nationally recognized for his accomplishments in the areas of healthcare, health literacy, cultural competency, diversity, ethics, patient's rights, safety and advocacy. He served as the Clinical Manager of the Clinical Ethics Center at Oakwood and later went on to become the Director of the Clinical Language Service. He was awarded Corp Magazine's Diversity Business Leader Award, Michigan Health Council's *Building Michigan's Healthcare Workforce Award*, and Oakwood's Service Excellence program of the year. Moe is board certified in healthcare administration and has taught courses in US healthcare systems and disparities at Eastern Michigan University. In 2011 he was named the Arab American of the Year in medicine. Moe has always professed that it was Gail Daly who was his mentor and the springboard for what went on to accomplish professionally.

Leonard Weber, PhD

Leonard Weber worked for over 40 years as an ethicist in the Detroit area, teaching at the University of Detroit Mercy and providing professional ethics services in a variety of healthcare organizations, including Oakwood, Beaumont, and Henry Ford. He was in the first generation of professional ethicists to work in hospitals, often assisting in the establishment of hospital Ethics Committees and in the education of their members.

Dr. Weber has written four books, including *Business Ethics In Healthcare*, and many articles. Following the completion of his Ph.D., from McMaster University in Ontario, he lived for over 50 years as a resident of the city of Detroit.

Chris (Christine) Westphal, NP, MSN, ACNS, ACHPN, FOCN

Chris Westphal retired after almost 50 years in nursing which included roles as a critical care nurse, Family Matters Support Service Clinical Nurse Specialist, researcher, educator, nurse leader, consultant and culminated in 18 years as a palliative care nurse practitioner. She has authored several articles, co-authored the award-winning *My Voice - My Choice* advance directive, and presented nationally on topics related to critical and palliative care. Currently Chris' focus is on spending time with family and friends but also continues to volunteer for the Hospice & Palliative Nurses Association (HPNA), serve as a peer reviewer for several journals and consult. A special interest is advocating for tissue/eye donation in hospice and palliative care. She played an instrumental role in the formation of Family Matters Support Service and the advancement of the Clinical Ethics Consultation Service.

Mary Catherine Wright, MSN, RN

Mary Catherine is a native Detroiter with over 42 years of working as a nurse. Mary Catherine was an Oakwood ethics committee member for many years. She developed and was the singular Family Matters staff at Oakwood Hospital's Taylor Michigan site for over 10 years, where she also helped develop their palliative care program. Her professional background includes educator, hospice nurse, and nursing administrative roles. She is a volunteer Parish Nurse at Saint Charles in Detroit and works collaboratively with Corewell Health's Community Department to bring health programs to St Charles. Mary Catherine continues her spiritual development and is currently in an 18-month discernment process for the Secular Franciscan Order. She attained a BSN from Oakland University in Rochester and MSN in Nursing Administration from the University of Michigan Ann Arbor.

The Authors

Ann Caulfield-Cook and Martha Hnatiuk have worked together in the clinical setting, the community setting, and through their advance directive consulting business. Most importantly, they collaborated closely with Gail Daly to bring *Closing the Circle* to life.

Ann Caulfield-Cook, PhD, LMSW

Dr. Caulfield-Cook is a retired clinical social worker. She received her PhD from the Institute for Clinical Social Work in Chicago and her MSW degree from the University of Michigan. She worked in the mental health field for 40 years. She had a private psychotherapy practice for 20 years before retiring in 2019.

In addition to her private practice, in 2008, she accepted a part-time position at Oakwood Hospital as the Social Work Supervisor in the Care Management Department. In 2012 she accepted the position of the Clinical Ethics Consultation Services Supervisor, wherein she managed the department budget, consult referrals, and the administrative duties of the System Clinical Ethics Committee.

Alongside her clinical work, she taught clinical social work courses at Wayne State University's School of Social Work and served as a faculty advisor to master's students in their field placement.

Ann resides in Allen Park with her husband and black lab, Boomer. Since retirement, she has become an avid pickleball player.

Martha Hnatiuk, MA, RN

Martha Hnatiuk is a retired RN and educator. She graduated from Bronson School of Nursing and began her career as a floor nurse at Oakwood Hospital in Dearborn, Michigan. She later went on to obtain her Master of Arts with a major in philosophy from Wayne State University in Detroit. She subsequently taught critical thinking at Wayne State as well as healthcare ethics for the University of Detroit-Mercy.

Martha took a position as a clinical nurse specialist for Family Matters and the Clinical Ethics Consultation Service in 2005. During her 10 years there, she gave numerous presentations throughout SE Michigan on the topic of advance directives and co-authored an updated version of the *My Voice - My Choice* advance directive packet.

Martha resides in Dearborn and enjoys the family cottage in Manistee, Michigan, a gathering place for sunset viewing and memory making with family and friends.